Edited by E.I. Hernández-Jiménez, E.M. Rakhanskaya

LASERS

IN COSMETIC DERMATOLOGY & SKINCARE PRACTICE

Cosmetics & Medicine
Publishing

Author/Editor:

Elena I. Hernández-Jiménez, *Ph.D.*

Editor:

Ekaterina M. Rakhanskaya, *M.D.*, neurologist, radiation safety specialist

Contributors:

Natalia G. Kalashnikova, *M.D.*, surgeon, dermatologist, laser therapist

Diana S. Urakova, *M.D., Ph.D.*, dermatologist, laser therapist

Alisa A. Sharova, *M.D., Ph.D.*, Associate Professor, dermatologist, gerontologist

Oleg V. Sheptii, *M.D.*, surgeon, dermatologist, laser therapist

Yuri M. Militch, hardware engineer

LASERS IN COSMETIC DERMATOLOGY AND SKINCARE PRACTICE

Much has been written about lasers, but only a few books cover laser cosmetic dermatology from beginning to end. We decided to address this gap and collected all the information that would be useful for specialists in this book. It focuses on modern laser and photodynamic technologies and deals in detail with various issues concerning high-energy and low-intensity devices.

The book consists of three parts. In the first part, we explain the nature of laser radiation and provide a general understanding of how a laser device is constructed. A separate chapter is devoted to the interaction of laser radiation with the skin — the targets and mechanisms of laser action and the essence of photothermolysis. This part also considers the features of intense pulse light (IPL) treatment, low-level laser therapy (LLLT), and photodynamic therapy (PDT).

The second part is devoted to practical issues — the specific capabilities of light-based and photodynamic technologies. The entire spectrum of dermatological and aesthetic problems in which lasers and IPL devices yield significant results are considered. These are laser rejuvenation, removal of benign growths, treatment of vascular and pigmentation disorders, scars, acne, psoriasis, and onychomycosis, as well as tattoo, unwanted hair (epilation), and fat deposit removal. In this part, we also discuss the current perspectives on the combination of laser treatment and injectable procedures, and the possibilities of using lasers for the transdermal delivery of active ingredients. A separate chapter on complications associated with laser procedures and ways to reduce their risks concludes the second part.

The third part touches on some key organizational aspects, such as requirements for safe operation and the choice of laser devices.

ISBN 978-1-970196-21-4 (paperback)

ISBN 978-1-970196-40-5 (hardcover)

ISBN 978-1-970196-14-6 (eBook — Adobe PDF)

ISBN 978-1-970196-38-2 (eBook — ePUB)

© Cosmetics & Medicine Publishing LLC, 2024

© Cover photo: VGstockstudio / Shutterstock

FirstEditing

English version is edited and certified by the FirstEditing.Com, Inc. (USA).

Author/Editor

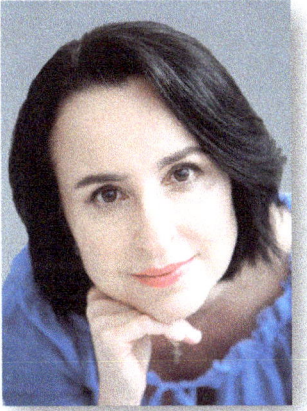

Elena I. Hernández-Jiménez, *Ph.D.*

Biophysicist, scientific journalist

Editor-in-chief of Cosmetics and Medicine Publishing

Chairperson of the Executive Board of the International Society of Applied Corneotherapy (I.A.C.)

Author and co-author of numerous publications in professional magazines, co-author and editor of the book series *Fundamentals of Cosmetic Dermatology & Skincare, Cosmetic Dermatology & Skincare Practice, Cosmetic Chemistry for Dermatology & Skincare Specialists* and others

Speaker at international conferences, author of training seminars and webinars for professionals in the field of skincare

Professional interests: biology and physiology of the skin, skin permeability, cosmetic chemistry, anti-age medicine, physiotherapy in dermatology and aesthetic medicine, skin analysis and imaging

Table of Contents

PART II
PRACTICAL SKILLS & CLINICAL EXPERIENCE

PART III
ORGANIZATIONAL MATTERS

Abbreviations

AEL	—	accessible emission limits
ALA	—	aminolevulinic acid
ALEX	—	alexandrite laser
ASDS	—	American Society for Dermatologic Surgery
ATP	—	adenosine triphosphate
BTA	—	botulinum toxin type A
CAD	—	capillary angiodysplasia
cAMP	—	cyclic adenosine monophosphate
DNA	—	deoxyribonucleic acid
ENT	—	ear, nose, and throat
Er:glass	—	erbium glass laser
Er:YAG	—	erbium-doped yttrium aluminum garnet laser
Er:YSGG	—	erbium, chromium:yttrium-scandium-gallium-garnet
FDA	—	U.S. Food and Drug Administration
GRADE	—	Grading of Recommendations, Assessment, Development and Evaluation
HA	—	hyaluronic acid
HIFU	—	high-intensity focused ultrasound
IL	—	interleukin
IPL	—	intense pulsed light
IR	—	infrared
KTP	—	potassium-titanyl-phosphate laser
LED	—	light-emitting diode
LLLR	—	low-level laser radiation
LLLT	—	low-level laser (light) therapy
MASER	—	Microwave Amplification by Stimulated Emission of Radiation
MLA	—	methyl aminolevulinic acid
MMP	—	matrix metalloproteinase
MPE	—	Maximum Permissible Exposure
mRNA	—	matrix ribonucleic acid
MTZ	—	microthermal zone
Nd:YAG	—	neodymium yttrium-aluminum-garnet laser

PDC	— pulse duration control
PDL	— pulsed dye laser
PDT	— photodynamic therapy
PPE	— personal protective equipment
QS	— Q-Switched
RF	— radiofrequency
ROS	— reactive oxygen species
RTD	— residual thermal damage
RUBY	— ruby laser
SMA	— spatially modulated ablation
SMAS	— superficial musculo-aponeurotic system
SPF	— sun protection factor
TAE	— telangiectasia
TGF-β	— transforming growth factor-beta
TNF-α	— tumor necrosis factor-alpha
TRT	— thermal relaxation time
UHF	— ultrahigh-frequency
UV	— ultraviolet
UVA	— ultraviolet type A
UVB	— ultraviolet type B
UVC	— ultraviolet type C

Part I

Theoretical basis

Chapter 1
Physics of laser radiation

To understand lasers and how they work, we must first understand light — the active factor in all light-based methods.

1.1. The nature of light

Light is electromagnetic radiation emitted by heated or excited matter. In everyday life, we consider light to be what we can see with our eyes — the visible range of the electromagnetic spectrum — but this is a very small part of it (**Fig. I-1-1**). The electromagnetic spectrum includes various types of electromagnetic radiation, differing from each other in frequency, wavelength, and power of the transferred energy, which will determine the properties and peculiarities of their interaction with biological tissues.

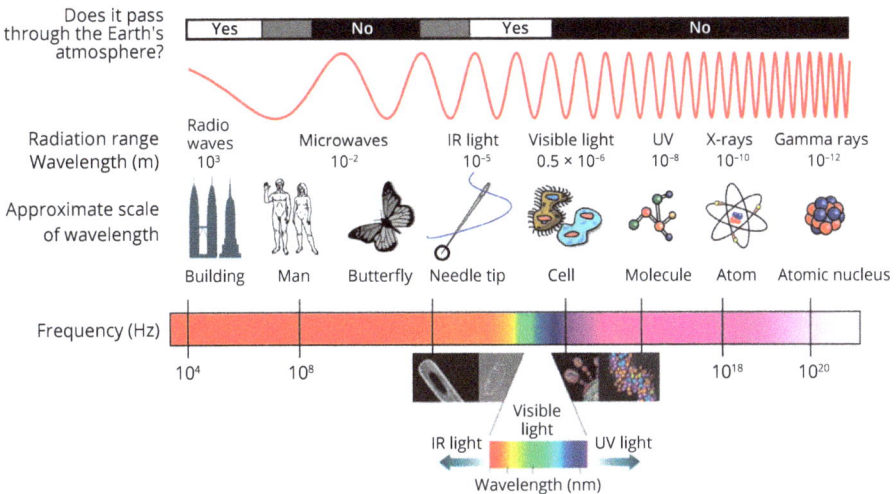

Figure I-1-1. Scale of electromagnetic oscillations

Electromagnetic radiation is an interconnected oscillation of electric and magnetic fields that make up a single electromagnetic field that propagates trough space in the form of waves. On this basis, in a very simplified form:

- **The frequency of electromagnetic radiation (υ)** is the number of electromagnetic wave crests that pass a reference point (observer, detector, etc.) in one second. Frequency is measured in hertz (Hz); 1 Hz is equivalent to one oscillation per second, while 1 megahertz (MHz) corresponds to one million oscillations per second.
- **The wavelength (λ)** is the distance between two neighboring wave crests, which is measured in units of length (nm, mm, etc.) (**Table I-1-1**).

Table I-1-1. Spectral bands of optical radiation

RADIATION	WAVELENGTH
Ultraviolet (UV)	**100–400 nm**
Ultraviolet type C (UVC), short-wave	100–280 nm
Ultraviolet type B (UVB), mid-wave	280–315 nm
Ultraviolet type A (UVA), long-wave	315–400 nm
Visible (optical)	**400–760 nm**
Infrared (IR)	**760 nm to 2000 μm**
Near-IR	760 nm to 2.5 μm (0.76–2.5 μm)
Mid-IR	2.5–50 μm
Far-IR	50–2000 μm

Electromagnetic radiation corresponding to the infrared (IR), visible (Vis), ultraviolet (UV), and X-ray ranges is the active factor in light-based medical technologies; the first three types are used in dermatology and aesthetic medicine. Low-intensity long-wave X-rays (0.1–0.25 nm) are used in superficial X-ray therapy (Buckeye therapy) to treat skin pathologies such as keloid scars.

1.2. Laser radiation

Laser is an acronym for **L**ight **A**mplification by **S**timulated **E**mission of **R**adiation.

The starting point in the creation of lasers is the work of Albert Einstein, who in 1916 not only promulgated his famous theory of relativity but also presented to the scientific community the concept of induced radiation, which is the basis for the creation of lasers. The theory of relativity was preceded by a discovery that, when an electron transitions from the upper (higher-energy) orbital in an atom to a lower-energy orbital, the energy difference between these electron levels is emitted as photons characterized by a certain frequency/wavelength.

The physical basis of laser operation is stimulated (induced) emission. The essence of this phenomenon is that an excited atom can emit a photon under the action of another photon without its absorption if the energy of the latter is equal to the energy difference between the atomic levels before and after the emission. In this case, the emitted photon is coherent to the photon that caused the emission (its "exact copy"). This is how Light Amplification by Stimulated Emission of Radiation (the meaning behind LASER) occurs. As a result, a weak light flux in the laser medium is amplified, not chaotically, but in one predetermined direction. Hence, we can get an "amplified" light flux with predictable characteristics (Eichler H.J. et al., 2018).

1.3. Lasers in dermatology

Even though the theoretical foundations had been laid, the practical realization of Einstein's ideas, as well as those of many other famous physicists (Paul Dirac, Louis de Broglie, etc.) came only "thanks" to World War II, when research in the field of ultra-high radiofrequencies led to the development of radio spectroscopy, oscillation theory, and ultra-high frequency (UHF) electronics, creating the basis for the development of fundamentally new devices — lasers.

In the early 1950s, Nikolai Basov, Alexander Prokhorov (Lebedev Physical Institute), and Charles Hard Townes from Columbia University (USA) independently developed the first molecular generator operating on ammonia vapor. Upon receiving induced radiation, the device amplified the microwaves passing through it, giving rise to the MASER (Microwave Amplification by Stimulated Emission of Radiation) concept. Soon after, a maser operating on a beam of hydrogen molecules was created.

The work with light waves followed. During 1957–1958, based on the results of active scientific communication with Charles Townes, Gordon Gould prepared drawings of an optical maser for the U.S. Patent Office and suggested a name for the new technology — LASER — given that it aimed to allow amplification of light waves by induced radiation. The new term was announced at a conference in 1959 and eventually became standard. The world's first real working ruby laser (RUBY) was presented by Theodore Maiman in 1960, who is considered the creator of lasers.

In 1961, Soviet scientists published the first academic article describing the creation and testing of a ruby laser unit. In the same year, the scientific community learned about the laser based on yttrium-aluminum garnet with neodymium (Nd:YAG). In 1962, the first argon laser was created, and the carbon dioxide (CO_2) laser was introduced in 1964.

The Meiman laser was not yet relevant to medicine, but in 1961, *Nature Magazine* published the first results of using such a device for retina photocoagulation. The first dermatologist to use the laser for aesthetic purposes was Leon Goldman, the "father" of laser medicine. In 1963, he publicized the results of using a RUBY laser with a wavelength of 694 nm to affect pigmented skin and hair follicles; in 1965, he proposed its use for tattoo removal. However, the U.S. Food and Drug Administration (FDA) did not approve the use of RUBY for hair removal because of technical problems with its precise focus. Goldman was not discouraged and continued his research in this direction, as a part of which he studied the interaction of laser radiation with biological tissues, as well as the safe use of laser facilities (Nouri K., 2012).

The dangers of using lasers — certain technical problems and high risk of scarring — limited their use in medicine for a long time. This finally changed when a truly revolutionary milestone was reached with the development of the **selective photothermolysis** concept by Richard Rox Anderson and John Parrish in 1983 (Anderson R.R., Parrish J.A., 1983).

Since the early 1980s, lasers have been used to correct age-related changes. The first procedures were performed with ablative CO_2 lasers, which became the "gold standard" of laser skin rejuvenation. For years, a continuous laser beam was used for "laser resurfacing" irrespective of the skin structures (epidermis and/or dermis) exposed to the radiation. Despite their effectiveness in correcting age-related changes, such procedures were associated with a long rehabilitation period (up to several weeks), pain, and various adverse side effects such as persistent erythema, post-inflammatory hypo- and hyperpigmentation, and scarring. In the mid-1990s, a more gentle and predictable erbium laser was introduced, which somewhat compensated for the disadvantages of CO_2 lasers, but also gave less pronounced results.

A kind of "optimization" of traumatic laser resurfacing was achieved in 2003, when Richard R. Anderson and Dieter Manstein proposed the concept of **fractional photothermolysis** (Manstein D. et al., 2004). Fractional treatment forms numerous microchannels surrounded by undamaged tissue. This reduces skin traumatization and, consequently, shortens the rehabilitation period. Due to a lower risk of side effects and complications, treatment could be done in wider application areas. The first device that implemented this principle was a non-ablative fiber-optic erbium laser with a wavelength of 1550 nm — Fraxel® (Reliant Technologies, USA, currently owned by Solta Medical, Inc., USA), which appeared on the market in 2004.

1.4. Principles of laser operation

Lasers are optical quantum generators that convert an initial energy flow (light, electric, thermal, chemical) into a laser beam. Their basis is an **active medium** — the substance exposed to external energy that produces stimulated emission (Eichler H.J. et al., 2018).

Before switching on the laser, all quantum systems (atoms/molecules) of its active medium are stable — electrons occupy a stable position on their basic orbitals. When energy is supplied, the so-called **pumping process** occurs — its absorption by the laser medium and the transition of electrons within the atoms/molecules of this medium to higher orbitals (energy levels). Since this state is extremely unstable, some atoms can spontaneously transition to a stable state whereby an electron will return to the main orbital. The excess energy resulting from this process will be released in the form of a quantum of light, which, having reflected from special mirrors (optical resonator), will again return to the laser working medium. Here, the mechanism of forced emission is triggered. As noted above, such a photon induces the transition of neighboring atoms from the excited to the stable state with the emission of completely identical photons. As the original photon is not absorbed, it continues to affect other excited atoms of the medium, as well as the newly formed photons (**Fig. I-1-2**).

The active medium of the laser is in a resonator — a structure with two mirrors affixed to opposite walls facing each other. One of these mirrors (the rear one) reflects the entire stream of generated photons, while the second one can partially transmit (**Fig. I-1-3**). Through a series of multiple reflections, a sufficient number of photons is accumulated

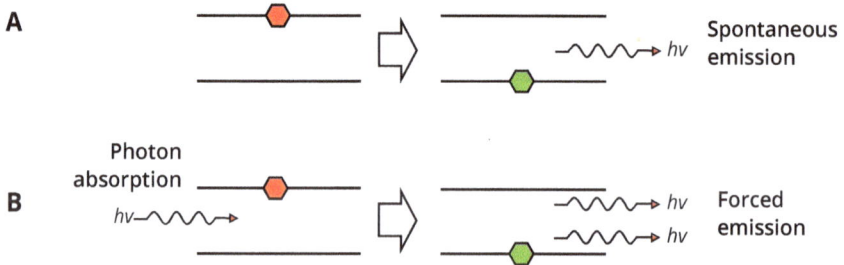

Figure I-1-2. Types of radiation: A — spontaneous; B — forced

h — Planck's constant, a fundamental universal constant that defines the quantum nature of energy and relates the energy of a photon to its frequency; v — photon frequency.

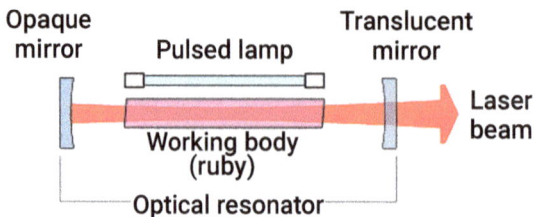

Figure I-1-3. Schematic diagram of a solid-state RUBY laser

to "break through" the front mirror. As a result, a common laser beam with completely identical emission characteristics is formed — and the greater the number of electrons returning to their ground levels, the more powerful it will be.

1.5. Basic characteristics of laser radiation

Lasers can create a radiation stream with unique monochromaticity, coherence, and collimation properties.

- **Monochromaticity.** All electromagnetic waves emitted by the laser have the same wavelength, for example, 694-nm RUBY, 2940-nm Er:YAG (erbium-doped yttrium aluminum garnet laser), 2790-nm Er:YSGG (erbium, chromium:yttrium-scandium-gallium-garnet), etc. Due to the high degree of monochromaticity, laser radiation has a high **spectral density**. That is, there is an increased concentration of light energy at one wavelength. This provides the necessary power of exposure as well as increases the accuracy of hitting the absorption peak of the target chromophore.
- **Coherence.** As laser radiation arises due to induced transitions of electrons from the upper level of the quantum system to the lower one, electromagnetic oscillations are synchronized in phase — the waves propagate as if "in sync." This provides maximum focusing of the laser.
- **Collimation.** High coherence reduces the angle of divergence of the laser beam to the limits determined by diffraction and thus increases the degree of directivity of the laser light source. Accordingly, the laser outputs a parallel beam of light that does not scatter with distance. This allows high brightness and maximum energy to be focused on the target.

1.6. Basic parameters of laser radiation

The following factors are considered the main physical parameters determining the peculiarities of laser action on biological tissues (Farkas J.P. et al., 2013):

- Emission wavelength
- Energy density (fluence) and power
- Duration and mode (pulsed or continuous) of irradiation
- Light spot size and the ability to focus the energy

1.6.1. Emission wavelength

The wavelength (λ) of laser radiation is determined by its active medium and it correlates with the peculiarities of the emitted light's absorption by individual skin structures. A specific absorption spectrum characterizes each substance; an absorption curve shows which types of radiation this substance (commonly called chromophore) absorbs more intensively, and which are absorbed less. Thus, by selecting a certain wavelength depending on the absorption spectrum of skin chromophores, we can target some of its individual structures.

The wavelength also determines the depth of light penetration into the skin: **the longer the wavelength, the deeper the penetration of light radiation into the skin**. IR rays penetrate tissues to a depth of up to 7 cm, while visible light penetrates up to 1 cm, and UV rays can reach 0.5–1.0 mm below the skin surface (**Table I-1-2**; **Fig. I-1-4**). In this case, the wavelength is inversely proportional to the energy of light quanta. This means that short-wavelength radiation has more energy than a long-wavelength laser beam.

Table I-1-2. Spectral bands of optical radiation and their penetration depth into the skin

SPECTRAL BAND	SKIN PENETRATION DEPTH (PHOTONS PENETRATING TO A GIVEN DEPTH, %)
UVC	30 µm (5%)
UVB	30 µm (33%)
UVA	30 µm (50%)
Colored stripes: from purple to red	1 mm (blue) (50%) 10 mm (red) (60%)
Near-IR	30–40 mm (60%)
Far-IR	

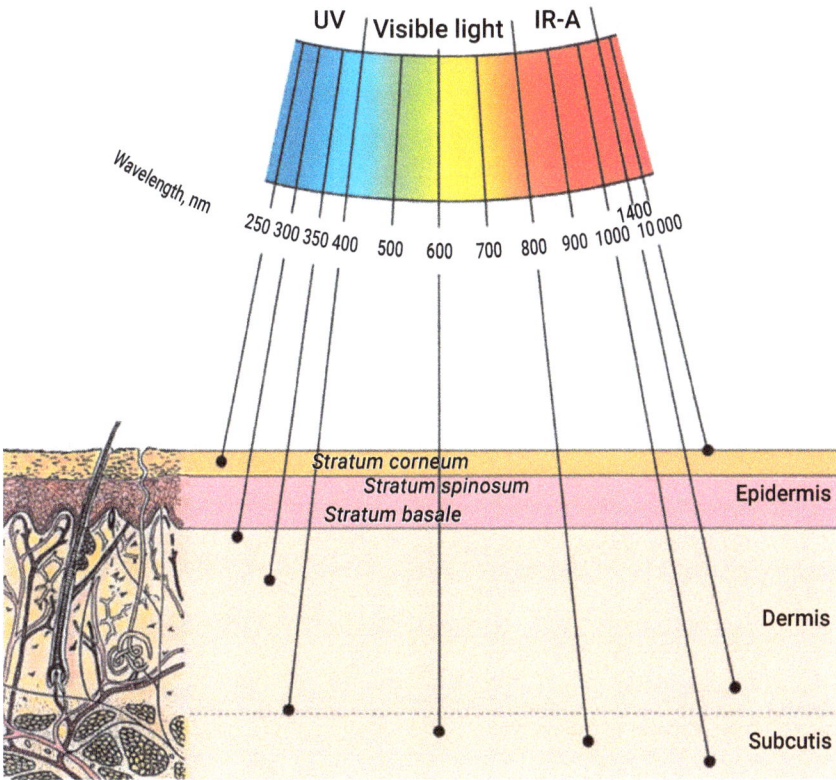

Figure I-1-4. Depth of light penetration as a function of the emission wavelength

Therefore, if we want to damage some specific skin structures, we need to consider both the absorption peaks of the target chromophores and the depth of the structures containing them when selecting laser treatment options.

1.6.2. Energy density (fluence) and power

How pronounced the effect on the chromophore will be and what impact it will have on the target structure depends on the energy (J) of the laser radiation and its power (W), which characterizes the rate of this energy input. In practice, these parameters are converted to energy density (fluence) (J/cm^2) and power density (energy flux density) (W/cm^2).

The amount of light energy in the radiation flux is characterized by its power (total energy carried by light per unit of time through a given surface) or light intensity (I), which is the power calculated per unit of surface perpendicular to which the light rays fall. The effects are usually normalized by the dose (**D**) of radiation, which is equal to the product of the light intensity (**I**) and the duration (**t**) of irradiation:

$$D = I \cdot t$$

It is important to remember that only the absorbed dose has a biological effect since the skin reflects part of the light. Specifically, the skin reflects about 60% of IR rays, 40% of visible light, and 10% of UV rays. For UV and Vis rays, the reflectivity of unpigmented skin is almost twice as high as that of pigmented skin. In the infrared region, the reflectivity of light-colored skin is about 20% higher.

In terms of radiation power, medical lasers are divided into:

- Low-power lasers: 1–5 mW
- Mid-power lasers: 6–500 mW
- High-power (high-intensity) lasers: over 500 mW

Low- and mid-power lasers belong to the so-called **biostimulating lasers (low-intensity lasers)**.

High-power lasers are used for photodestructive treatments. The specific effects will depend on the radiation's power density, i.e., the power per 1 cm². Namely, dissection is performed in the 50–100 W/cm² range, and vaporization of soft tissues occurs in the 500–850 W/cm² range.

1.6.3. Irradiation duration and mode (pulsed or continuous)

Ideally, when working with a laser, we want to deliver an amount of energy to the target structure that will cause it damage but will leave non-target tissues intact. Therefore, the target must have time to cool down between energy delivery pulses, as otherwise heat will spread beyond the target to the neighboring areas.

The time required for this cooling will depend on the skin structure and is determined by the **thermal relaxation time (TRT)** for a given target (**Table I-1-3**). TRT is the period required to transfer

Table I-1-3. Thermal relaxation time (TRT)

STRUCTURE	SIZE, μm	TRT
Tattoo pigment	0.5–4	20 ns
Melanosoma	0.1–0.5	250 ns
Hair follicle	200	18 ms
Erythrocyte (hemoglobin as chromophore)	7.5–8.3	2 μs
Vessels	50	1.2 ms
	100	4.8 ms
	200	19 ms
	300	42.6 ms
	Leg veins	Up to 100 ms
Epidermis	Thickness of 27.8–34.6	5–10 ms

63% of the heat received (e = 2.7-fold reduction in thermal energy) to the surrounding tissues (Murphy M.J., Torstensson P.A., 2014).

The irradiation mode relates to the emission mode, which can be continuous, quasi-continuous, or pulsed. The latter option avoids undesirable overheating and damage to non-target structures due to tissue cooling between pulses (**Fig. I-1-5**). If the energy transfer duration to the chromophore (pulse duration) is higher than its TRT or the interval between pulses is reduced, heat will spread beyond the target, which may lead to undesirable overheating of neighboring structures.

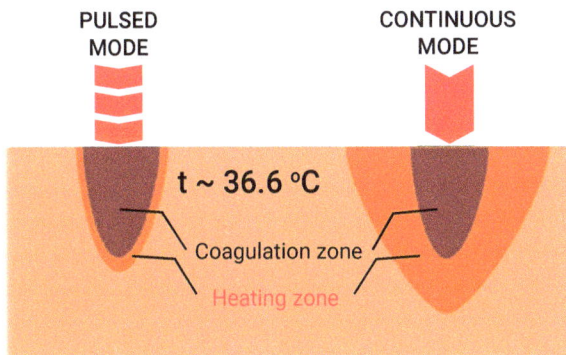

Figure I-1-5. Tissue impact area when using continuous and pulsed modes

Modern laser systems use special patented technologies to generate laser pulses that range from ultra-short to ultra-long. The longer the pulse duration, the more pronounced the photothermal effect and the predominance of coagulation over ablation will be (this applies to long-pulsed lasers in particular). The shorter the pulse duration, the greater the precision and the more likely it is to achieve the photoacoustic effect (see Part I, section 2.2.2).

Q-switched (QS) technology is used today to generate powerful pulses of nanosecond (ns) and even picosecond (ps) duration (passive QS technology) to obtain ultra-short pulses. For this purpose, during laser pumping, the optical resonator properties are intentionally "degraded" via various approaches to prevent spontaneously generated photons from triggering the induced emission process. As this results in an excess of atoms in the excited state, the properties of the resonator are quickly "improved," and all the stored energy can be released in the form of a short, powerful pulse. In a variant of this design used in lasers for hair or tattoo removal, QS pulses are split into pulse trains (a sequence of lower-energy QS pulses). This energy delivery method is believed to avoid the formation of powerful acoustic waves that can traumatize non-target skin structures. Mode-locking is another technology for producing ultra-short pulses, such as those of ps and femtosecond (fs) duration. To summarize, different technologies can be used in ultra-short pulse lasers, allowing the production of high-power pulses of very short duration.

When operating in pulsed mode, the pulse repetition rate must be carefully selected, as it sets the rate at which the pulses are emitted. The pulse repetition rate is measured in pulses per second, or hertz (Hz).

Another critical parameter for laser operation is the pulse shape. For example, the **pulse duration control (PDC) system** in Sharplight laser for photoepilation facilitates control of the pulse configuration. In this case, the beam can be emitted in one of the following PDC modes (**Fig. I-1-6**):

- **Smooth pulse:** Rectangular, uniform pulses with low peak power and a delayed heating effect are formed. This mode is used for skin phototypes I–V and is ideal for dark skin, thick dark hair, and sun-damaged or aging skin.

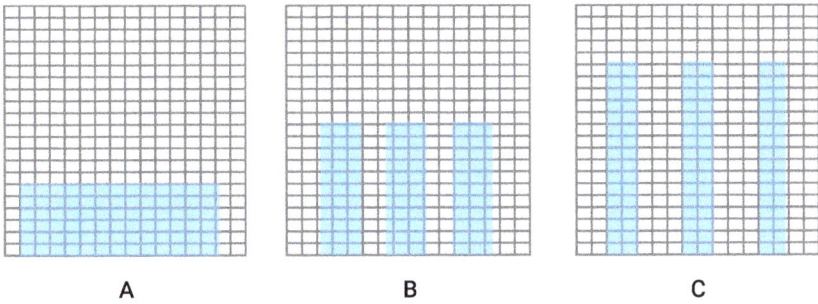

Figure I-1-6. Dynamic pulse control modes: A — smooth pulse; B — long pulse; C — high pulse

- **Long pulse:** Pulses with a 50% fill factor, with equal 'on' and 'off' intervals. Designed for skin phototypes I–IV and for brown hair of medium thickness.
- **High pulse (hard pulse):** Pulses with high peak power. Intended for skin phototypes I–III, excellent for fair skin, and "fine blonde and russet hair.

The continuous mode of laser delivery, i.e., a continuous beam, is rarely used in modern dermatology, as its main application is the removal of various types of malformations and tissue dissection in surgery. When quasi-continuous modes are used in dermatology, the pump source is 'on' for intervals as short as necessary to reduce the effects associated with heat generation but still long enough for stable, almost continuous emission.

Q-switching is a technique by which a laser can produce a ns or ps pulsed output beam with extremely high peak power — much higher than would be produced by the same laser operating in a continuous mode. Today, QS lasers have largely replaced long-pulsed lasers and continuous-beam ablative treatments for pigment lesions, tattoo removal, and epilation.

1.6.4. Light spot and energy focusing

From the medical point of view, an important **spatial characteristic of a light beam is the small divergence of its rays, called collimation in physics**. The higher the divergence, the more difficult it is to collect rays in a small spot, which is often necessary for localized treatment, for example, in photoepilation. The practical relevance of collimation is best seen by comparing the area of light spots from a pocket flashlight and a laser pointer, with the latter producing parallel rays within a very narrow beam. This characteristic allows for good optical focusing and, thus, the high energy density of quanta (in other words, a high concentration of energy in a microscopically small volume of matter), as well as the possibility of transmitting radiation over long distances using light guides.

The size of the light spot also determines the effective depth of exposure, which is another important parameter. Since photon scattering occurs when laser radiation interacts with tissue, it limits the delivery of the necessary energy to deep chromophores, which is important, for example, in the case of hair removal or removal of vascular defects. A large spot can reduce scattering losses and direct more photons to the target structure, providing more profound and more efficient laser energy delivery. Conversely, if a superficial effect is desired, the spot size should be reduced (**Fig. I-1-7**).

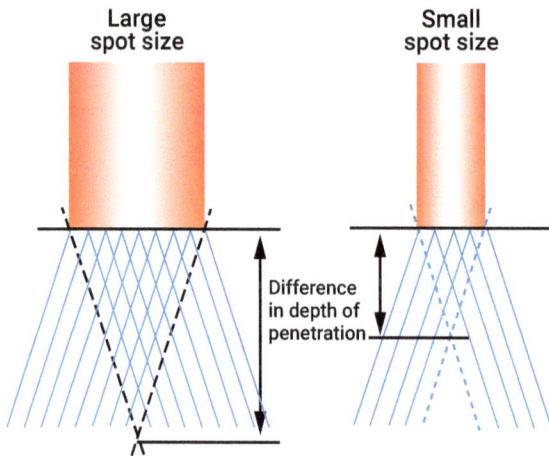

Figure I-1-7. Dependence of the effective penetration depth of radiation on the laser spot size

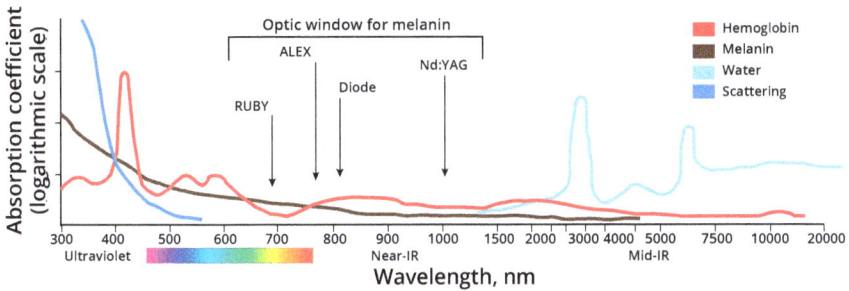

Figure I-1-8. Radiation spectrum of lasers used in dermatology and aesthetic medicine

1.6.5. Types of lasers

The wavelength and other parameters pertaining to laser radiation are determined by the properties of the laser working body — the material or medium that is pumped and forms the stimulated emission (**Fig. I-1-8**). Depending on the active medium, the following types of laser radiation sources are distinguished (**Table I-1-4**):

- **Liquid lasers:** The working medium consists of organic solvent and dye; this is the case for, for example, pulsed dye laser (PDL); the pumping is performed by a pulsed lamp or other laser.
- **Gas lasers:** The working medium consists of carbon dioxide, krypton, argon, or gas mixtures; pumped by electric discharges.
- **Excimer lasers:** Type of gas lasers based on electronic transitions of molecules existing only in the electronically excited state, i.e., argon–fluorine, krypton–chlorine, krypton–fluorine, etc.
- **Solid-state lasers:** Consisting of crystals or glass, where the solid material is enriched with chromium, erbium, neodymium, or titanium ions; pumped by a pulsed lamp or other lasers.
- **Semiconductor lasers:** Consisting of semiconductor crystals such as gallium arsenide (GaAs). The most typical example of a semiconductor laser are laser diodes, also made of semiconductor materials. The fundamental difference between semiconductor and solid-state lasers is that the stimulated emission in the former type is formed not by the transition of electrons between orbitals, but by transitions between energy zones or subzones of the crystal; pumping is performed by electric current.

Table I-1-4. Main characteristics of biomedical lasers

WORKING BODY	WAVELENGTH, nm	OPERATION MODE
Solid-state lasers		
Neodymium:YAG	1064/1320	Pulsed, continuous
Ruby	694	Pulsed
Alexandrite (ALEX)	720–780	Pulsed
Holmium:YAG	2100	Pulsed, continuous
Erbium fiber	1540/1550	Pulsed
Erbium:YSGG	2790	Pulsed
Erbium:YAG	2940	Pulsed
Gas lasers		
Helium–cadmium	325	Continuous
Nitrogen	337 (316/357)	Pulsed, continuous
Argon	488–514	Continuous
Helium–neon	554/594/663/1152	Continuous
Krypton	460–680	Continuous
Gold vapors	528	Continuous
	2600–3300	Continuous
Carbon dioxide	10,600	Pulsed, continuous
Liquid lasers		
Organic dye	300–900	Pulsed, continuous
Excimer lasers		
Argon–fluorine	193	Pulsed
Krypton–chlorine	222	Pulsed, continuous
Krypton–fluorine	248	Pulsed
Xenon–chlorine	308	Pulsed
Xenon–fluorine	351	Pulsed
Semiconductor lasers (laser diodes)		
Gallium arsenide	Red and IR spectrum	Pulsed
Aluminum gallium arsenide		Pulsed, continuous

Chapter 2
Interaction of laser radiation with skin

The interaction between the laser beam and the skin obeys the physical laws: laser light, like any light, can be reflected, scattered, absorbed, or simply pass through a medium (**Fig. I-2-1**).

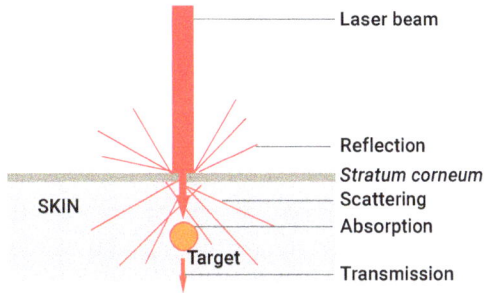

Figure I-2-1. Interaction of laser radiation with skin

2.1. Laser targets

We can significantly affect a medium only if it absorbs the laser energy. Obtaining additional energy by a molecule (transition to an excited state) can trigger physicochemical and biological reactions that form the final therapeutic effect. At the same time, each type of electromagnetic field and radiation causes photobiological processes inherent only to it, determining the specificity of their therapeutic effects.

Thus, light technologies are based on the specific interaction of electromagnetic radiation of a particular wavelength (photons) with specific substances in the skin that can absorb this radiation. These substances, called chromophores, are the main targets of irradiation.

Although any molecule is characterized by its light absorption features, the main chromophores for laser aesthetic treatment are (Anderson R.R., 2013; Han G., 2014):
■ Endogenous chromophores (those found naturally in the skin):
  – melanin

- hemoglobin (oxy- and deoxyhemoglobin)
- water
■ Exogenous chromophores (those applied to or introduced into the skin externally):
  - tattoo pigment
  - photosensitizers

Cosmetic particles are also exogenous chromophores, although we should avoid exposure to them.

Each chromophore is characterized by its absorption spectrum — a curve showing the intensity with which they absorb radiation of different wavelengths (**Fig. I-2-2**).

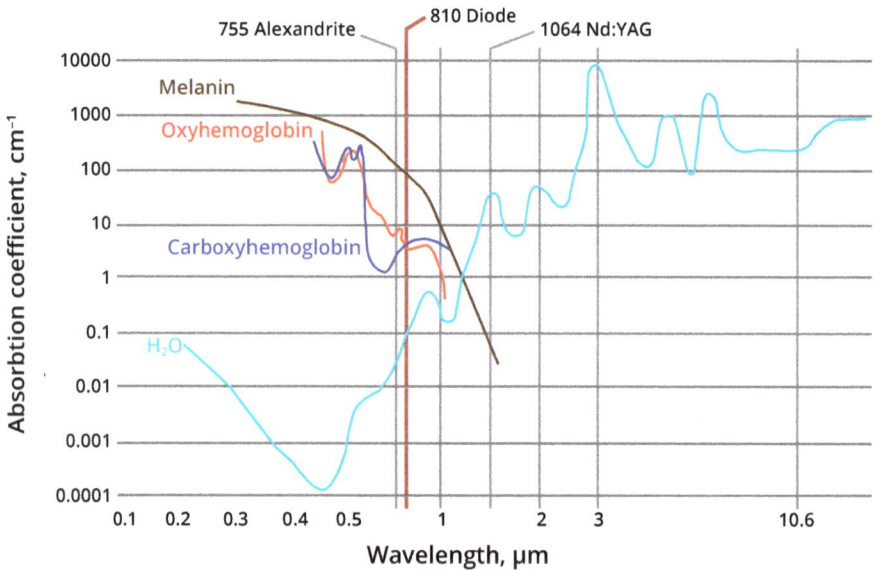

Figure I-2-2. Laser radiation absorption spectra of different skin chromophores

2.2. Mechanisms of laser action

Further events following the absorption of photons can develop according to different scenarios, but the first stage is always the same — the corresponding chromophores absorb photons.

In terms of physics, electromagnetic radiation energy is converted into other types of energy when it interacts with molecules in body tissues:

- **Chemical:** changing the configuration of electron bonds in the molecule and its reactivity
- **Thermal:** increasing the amplitude of oscillations of the molecule

Heating of the skin when its surface is irradiated occurs for two reasons:
1. Light absorption by chromophores (primary)
2. Light scattering on the optical inhomogeneities of the epidermis and dermis (secondary)

Even minor heating is fraught with serious consequences, as tissue damage may occur at relatively low temperatures — starting at 42–45 °C (**Table I-2-1**). In some cases, such as classical high-energy laser technologies, this is exactly what we desire, while in others (low-intensity laser treatment) we try to avoid it (Niemz M.H., 2019).

Table I-2-1. Tissue responses to heating by light exposure to different temperature

TEMPERATURE (°C)	BIOLOGICAL EFFECTS
42–45	Structural changes in proteins, hydrogen bond breakage, tissue retraction (tightening)
45–50	Inactivation of enzymes, gelatinization of lipids, changes in membrane permeability
50–60	Denaturation of proteins and DNA, closure of the vascular lumen
65–80	Collagen denaturation
100	Water boiling, rupture of vacuoles
100–300	Vaporization (ablation), fast
200	Elastin denaturation
100–300	Carbonization (after vaporization), slow

Depending on the intensity of laser exposure (energy, pulse duration, and other parameters), the following reactions can occur in irradiated tissues (Niemz M.H., 2019):

- Photothermal (heating by absorption of light energy)
- Photoacoustic (or photomechanical)
- Photochemical

Laser radiation can realize its effect on tissues due to a combination of mechanisms. For example, in the case of short-pulsed lasers, the shorter the pulse duration, the greater the contribution of photoacoustic destruction and the lesser the contribution of photothermal destruction.

2.2.1. Photothermal effect

As a result of light energy absorption, the chromophore molecules are heated and transfer heat to their surroundings. Depending on the degree of heating, the following variants of thermal tissue damage are possible (**Fig. I-2-3**):

- Coagulation ("gluing")
- Vaporization ("vaporization")
- Carbonization ("charring")

In medicine, tissue destruction by light is called **photothermolysis**. Depending on the chromophore, two variants of photothermolysis are distinguished.

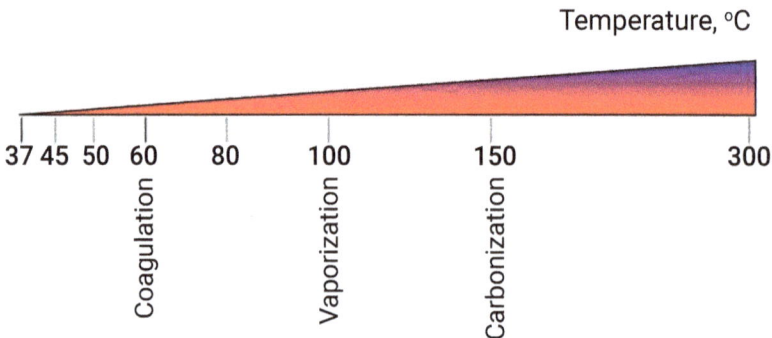

Temperature, °C

37 45 50 60   80   100   150   300

Coagulation   Vaporization   Carbonization

Figure I-2-3. Thermal effect of laser radiation on tissue

Non-selective photothermolysis

In non-selective photothermolysis, the target chromophore is water. As water is present in all living cells, its heating causes volumetric heating of the tissue (see Part I, section 2.4). For this purpose, laser devices emitting in the IR region are used: CO_2 (10,600 nm), Er:YAG (2940 nm) and Er:YSGG (2790 nm).

The following procedures are based on non-selective photothermolysis:

- Dissection (surgical laser scalpel)
- Laser resurfacing (layer-by-layer removal)
- Laser rejuvenation (fractional treatment)

Selective photothermolysis

Selective heating of various skin chromophores without significant water heating is possible (see Part I, section 2.3). This approach is realized with visible light sources and is used to affect:

- Vascular lesions (chromophore: hemoglobin)
- Pigmented structures such as hair and age spots (chromophore: hemoglobin)
- Adipocytes (chromophore: lipids)

Selectivity and efficiency of exposure to light of a specific wavelength can be increased by exogenous introduction of appropriate substances — chromophores with high absorption coefficients and the ability to accumulate in the area to be destroyed. This principle is the basis of **photodynamic therapy (PDT)** (Rkein A.M., Ozog D.M., 2014; Lee C.N. et al., 2020).

Selective photothermolysis exposes targets located deep in the skin with minimal traumatization of the barrier structures (the *stratum corneum*), facilitating rehabilitation.

2.2.2. Photoacoustic (photomechanical) effect

This mechanism is realized when a very large amount of energy is transferred to the chromophore over a very short time interval (in the ns and ps range). Such high-energy ultra-short pulses cause electrons to detach from chromophores, forming a rapidly expanding plasma cloud that eventually "explodes" with the formation of shock-waves. This is believed to lead to the formation of "optical breakdowns" accompanied by cavitation (forming cavities of 0.1–0.2 mm diameter) without residual thermal damage.

The photoacoustic effect is characteristic of picosecond lasers. It also appears when Er:YAG is operated in a special mode in which optical energy is converted into a mechanical wave propagating deep into the tissue. This transformation is called spatially modulated ablation (SMA) and is performed by the SMA module (Volkova N.V. et al., 2019). With its help, the light beam is scattered and causes microablation dots. The resulting acoustic waves propagate through the tissues to a depth of up to 6 mm, forming microshock and microdestruction areas with minimal skin surface damage. Microdamage in the skin's deep layers triggers regeneration, leading to remodeling of the dermis structure. Er:YAG + SMA can be used for skin rejuvenation and scar revision, providing a safer alternative to fractional CO_2 laser (Trelles M.A. et al., 2016).

2.2.3. Photobiomodulation

Photobiomodulation is characterized by exposure to low-intensity laser radiation (LLLR) in the red or near-infrared part of the spectrum. Such exposure does not cause damage to skin structures but triggers or inhibits various biophysical aspects of cellular activity, resulting in positive therapeutic effects (see Part I, chapter 4).

2.3. Selective photothermolysis

The earliest studies on laser effects on human skin demonstrated the ability of light to selectively affect specific skin structures. However, the embodiment of these observations in specific applied technologies became possible only after Richard Rox Anderson and John Parrish of the Wellman Center for Photomedicine at Harvard Medical School formulated the **principles of selective photothermolysis** (Anderson R.R., Parrish J.A., 1983).

Their idea was to apply a laser beam to a chromophore with a much higher concentration in the target cell. The light parameters (wavelength, intensity, and duration of irradiation) are selected considering the chromophore's absorption spectrum to transfer as much energy as possible to its molecules. After absorbing quanta of light, the chromophore enters an excited state. In contrast, the reverse transition is accompanied by the release of "excess" energy into the surrounding space in the form of heat. Thus, light-induced heating causes irreversible destruction of both the target cell and, if necessary, its immediate neighbors (**enhanced selective photothermolysis**).

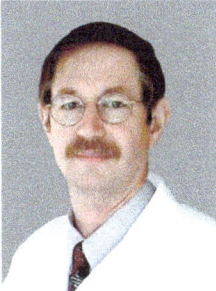

Richard Rocks Anderson

Modern technologies based on these selective photothermolysis principles rely on selective absorption of light by hemoglobin and melanin (as well as various exogenous chromophores), the absorption spectra of which are shown in **Fig. I-2-2**. By using radiation characterized by a suitable wavelength and other parameters, we can target areas of chromophore accumulation.

For dermatological treatments based on selective photothermolysis, laser and non-laser (intense pulsed light, IPL) light sources emitting in the 400–1200 nm wavelength range are used.

The following basic conditions must be met to realize a valid selectivity of exposure:

1. **Optical selectivity:** The chromophore of the target structure should have a higher absorption coefficient for radiation of a given wavelength than the chromophores in the surrounding tissues.
2. **Thermal selectivity:** The exposure duration should be equal to or lower than the target's TRT to ensure that the energy imparted by the light pulse to the biological object is expended on its heating and destruction but is not transferred to the surrounding tissues.
3. **Energy selectivity:** Sufficient energy is needed to destroy the target.

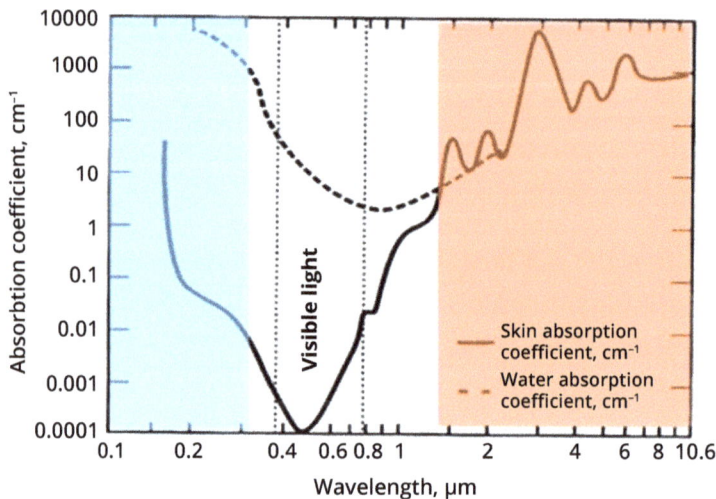

Figure I-2-4. Absorption spectra of tissue and water

2.4. Non-selective photothermolysis

Despite its name, non-selective photothermolysis is also a selective process. In this case, the chromophore will be water, but because water is present in all cells, the effect will not be on some individual targets but on all cells, i.e., it will not be selective.

Non-selective photothermolysis is based on photoablation, the almost instantaneous vaporization of tissue at high temperatures. For ablation to occur, the tissue must be rapidly heated to several hundred degrees Celsius.

Fig. I-2-4 shows a plot of light absorption by tissue and water as a function of radiation wavelength. It is easy to see that the two spectra are correlated. Radiation from the far-IR and UV regions of the spectrum is best absorbed by the tissue, which means that its penetration depth will be minimal, and all light energy will be released as heat in a minimal tissue volume. Obviously, UV light cannot be used as a heating factor because it is dangerous in high doses. But far-IR light has no such contraindications, so this part of the spectrum is employed in ablative (i.e., ablation-inducing) methods. Such procedures are performed using CO_2, Er:YAG and Er:YSGG lasers, which are thus known

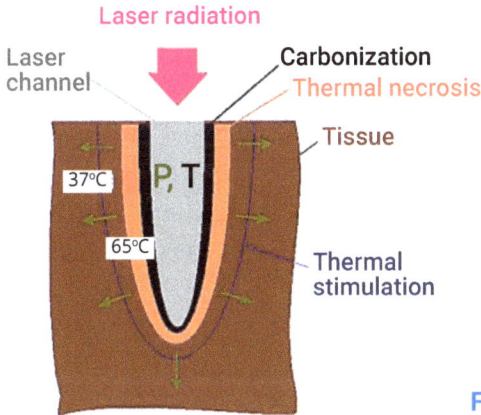

Figure I-2-5. Laser ablation

as **ablative lasers**. Water molecules also absorb near-IR radiation, although less actively — this is the radiation of Diode (1440 nm), Nd:YAG (1320, 1440 nm), Er:glass (1540 and 1550 nm), and Thulium (1927 nm) lasers. Their energy is not sufficient for ablation; they work through coagulation and are classified as **non-ablative**.

High-intensity IR radiation is absorbed mainly in the cell layers of the epidermis (at a depth of up to 50 μm). There will be practically no absorption in the *stratum corneum*, as its water content is low (10–30% of the total weight). The thermal effect will be the greatest in the layer of maximal absorption (within the optical depth of light penetration). The degree of temperature increase primarily depends on the radiation energy per unit area and the rate of temperature equalization between the heated and cold parts of the tissue. While ablation effects are observed in the zone of maximal absorption, other thermal effects such as charring, coagulation, or photobiological changes are possible in the boundary zone (characterized by downward temperature gradient) (**Fig. I-2-5**). The faster the heat dissipation, the more difficult it is to maintain the required high temperature in the zone of maximal absorption and the greater the radiation energy density required to heat the tissue.

The zone of thermal damage adjacent to the ablation zone is the zone of **residual thermal damage (RTD)**. If the laser pulse duration exceeds TRT, the heat spreads beyond the absorption region and the zone of boundary thermal damage increases.

Thermal effects depend on the energy density of the laser radiation. For ablation to occur, the energy density of the radiation must exceed a specific threshold value. If the ablation threshold is not reached, coagulation, vaporization, and charring will occur instead of tissue vaporization.

In cosmetic dermatology, non-selective photothermolysis is at the heart of procedures using continuous and fractionated laser beams.

2.4.1. Laser resurfacing

Laser resurfacing is an ablative procedure in which a continuous laser beam completely **vaporizes** and **coagulates** soft tissue at a certain depth (Boehm K.S. et al., 2020; Verma N. et al., 2023).

The first laser resurfacing procedure was performed in the early 1980s using a CO_2 laser (Yumeen S., Khan T., 2023). Accordingly, CO_2 laser can be rightly considered a pioneer in this field, and it has not lost its relevance to this day. Still, it should be recognized that the widespread use of CO_2 lasers for laser resurfacing is supported not so much by outstanding results, but by more prosaic reasons. These lasers are relatively cheap and are produced in many countries.

The first CO_2 lasers worked in continuous and long-pulsed mode, resulting in the tissue exposure duration that often exceeded several milliseconds (ms). During such a long period, the treated skin becomes very hot and transfers part of the heat to the neighboring areas. The treated tissue acquires a dark brown color and looks approximately the same, so it is difficult to visually control the degree of tissue damage, even for an experienced doctor. The ablation depth directly correlates with the number of passes performed and is usually limited to the epidermis. At the same time, a so-called "ablation plateau" commonly occurs, as the water content in the tissue decreases after the first pass, and ablation becomes less effective, but thermal damage increases. Since the skin is heterogeneous in thickness, repeated passes can extend the effects beyond the epidermis and can significantly damage the basal membrane and papillary dermis, resulting in scarring.

However, it should be noted that modern technologies are improving, and the impact is becoming more controlled. This advancement is due to the use of special scanning systems that guide the laser beam and prevent excessive passes or overlaps, as well as the reduction of pulse duration down to 1 ms ("superpulse" mode) and even less ("ultrapulse" mode). Such technologies allow shifting the damage from CO_2 lasers towards "pure" ablation, reducing the coagulation effect.

Er:YAG is superior to CO_2 lasers due to the greater predictability of results and more precise control (Yumeen S. et al., 2023). The operating wavelength of an Erbium laser is 2940 nm. Such radiation is absorbed by water 10 times more intensively than CO_2 laser radiation, so it is completely absorbed in the superficial layers of the skin.

In addition, as the pulses of light emitted by Erbium laser are short, all the energy is transferred to the upper layer of skin so quickly that it vaporizes before any energy can be transmitted to the surrounding tissue. Thus, with the help of Er:YAG, the top layer of skin can be carefully "removed" without overheating the deeper layers. Moreover, due to the absence of a coagulated layer, multiple passes can be performed, and the skin can be removed layer by layer to the desired level, although in most cases, Er:YAG is used for superficial procedures. The latest Er:YAG devices with variable-geometry rectangular pulse (VSP technology) provide pulses of variable duration, allowing the practitioner to select the laser exposure — from "cold" ablative peeling to deeper thermal coagulation (**Fig. I-2-6**).

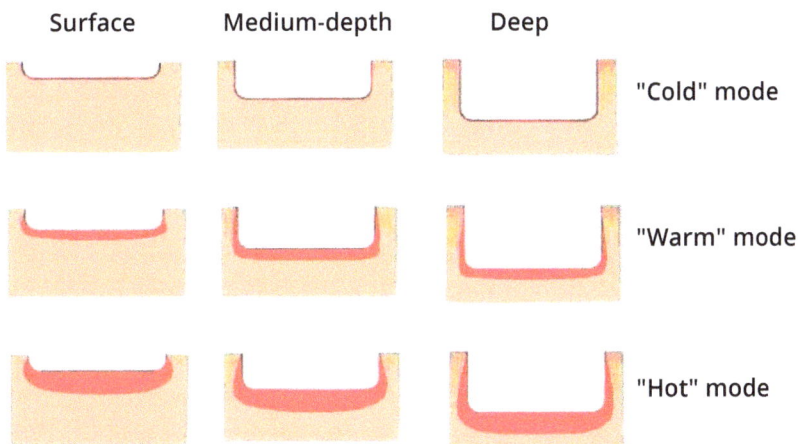

Figure I-2-6. Ablation and coagulation depth achieved by Er:YAG laser

Still, it should be noted that Er:YAG is more expensive than CO_2 laser; its average market price is about 70,000 EUR. Moreover, the "softness" of Erbium laser is both a plus and a minus. The undoubted benefit is the lower risk of complications, whereas the downside is that, after deep resurfacing with CO_2 laser the skin is better tightened than after Erbium laser treatment, and active remodeling processes are also initiated in the coagulation and thermal stimulation zones.

Adjustable laser beam penetration depth allows practitioners to work both at the level of the *stratum corneum* ("cold" laser peeling with Erbium laser is usually used for this purpose) and to affect the layers of the epidermis under the *stratum corneum* ("hot" laser peeling with CO_2 laser). Laser exposure allows jewelry-precision interventions aimed at small areas. The laser beam is ideal for peeling the skin around the eyes and lips, including their corners. Whereas "cold" laser peeling yields the effect of simple exfoliation (in the case of a small number of passes), "hot" laser peeling intensively warms the lower layers of the skin, and its effect builds up over 2–3 months.

The following disadvantages are common to CO_2 and Er:YAG lasers:

- Inability to perform procedures at times of increased solar activity due to the risk of hyperpigmentation
- Long rehabilitation period — from two weeks for Er:YAG to 2–3 months for CO_2 laser
- Visible demarcation line between the treated (on the face) and untreated (neck) areas due to the impossibility of carrying out treatments on the skin of the hands and neck
- Painful treatment (anesthesia is required)

2.4.2. Fractional photothermolysis

Fractional photothermolysis was proposed in 2003 as an alternative to laser resurfacing and non-ablative photorejuvenation with IPL systems by the creators of the selective photothermolysis concept Richard Rocks Anderson and Dieter Manstein (Manstein D. et al., 2004).

The idea of fractional laser treatment came to Dr. Anderson while reading a newspaper. He noticed that the pictures were printed in black, gray, and white dots. This prompted him to consider irradiating the skin not with a continuous stream of light, but with individual

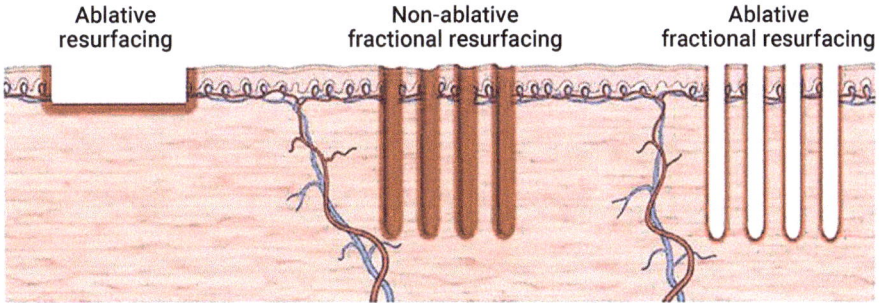

Figure I-2-7. Differences between laser resurfacing, ablative and non-ablative fractional laser treatment

microbeams forming pinpoint lesions in the skin. This is how the concept known as **fractional photothermolysis** came about, where volumetric heating is replaced by fractional heating. This treatment is much less traumatic, carrying fewer risks and expediting the recovery.

Microthermal treatment zones (MTZs) are formed in the process of skin exposure to the laser energy. These are zones of photothermolysis (ablation, coagulation), and their size depends on the beam diameter and energy (Laubach H.J. et al., 2006).

Depending on the radiation ranges used, two types of fractional photothermolysis are distinguished (**Fig. I-2-7**):

- **Ablative:** Light that is readily absorbed by water molecules is used (10,600-nm CO_2 laser and 2940-nm Er:YAG). Upon absorption, water is heated to 150–300 °C. The resulting steam instantly evaporates, and with it evaporate parts of cell walls and other structures of the epidermis and dermis (tissue vaporization). Even the *stratum corneum* is damaged despite its low water content.
- **Non-ablative:** Light that is relatively low absorbed by water molecules (in the 1300–2000 nm range) is used. Upon absorption, treated tissue heats up to 45–90 °C (coagulation) but the *stratum corneum* remains intact.

Currently, laser beam fractionation technologies are also used in lasers for selective photothermolysis.

The treatment field comprises thousands of isolated microthermal zones surrounded by intact tissue. Aseptic inflammation develops in the MTZ area, during which the debris of coagulated structures (microscopic epidermal necrotic debris) containing melanin, collagen, and elastin is partially evacuated through the MTZ channel in the epidermis and is partially captured and hydrolyzed by macrophages migrating to the inflammation zone. The basal layer of the epidermis recovers rather quickly, and exfoliation of the evacuated debris begins.

The proliferative stage of inflammation that develops at the MTZ site involves biosynthesizing new epidermal and dermal elements and reorganizing the surrounding tissue space. The MTZ healing process differs from other approaches because the intact skin areas between MTZs contain viable cells, including epidermal stem cells and fibroblasts.

The speed of re-epithelialization is directly proportional to the number and density of stem cells. Therefore, re-epithelialization of the treatment area is rapid, with minimal side effects. Damage-induced collagen retraction and remodeling ultimately lead to changes in the structure and mechanical properties of the dermis intercellular matrix, providing wrinkle smoothing and rejuvenation effects.

One of the main advantages of fractional laser therapy is that there are no open lesions, and the *stratum corneum* regains its integrity 24 hours after the procedure, and in the case of non-ablative treatment, it is not damaged at all. Thus, recovery is much faster than after laser resurfacing and complications such as dyschromia can be avoided. The risk of scarring is also reduced, allowing safe treatment of areas most prone to scarring, such as the neck and chest. A greater penetration depth can also be achieved as the skin surface is not ablated.

The MTZ depth for hypertrophic scars can be up to 4 mm. In conventional rejuvenation procedures, the depth is usually less than 1 mm.

Fractional lasers are used to eliminate fine lines and smooth deep wrinkles, enlarged pores, and atrophic scars (including post-acne), as well as restore skin structure, treat striae, achieve skin lifting (including upper and lower eyelids), and treat pigmentation disorders (melasma, solar and senile lentigo).

The high procedure efficiency, minimal rehabilitation period, ease of laser use, and lack of consumables make fractional photothermolysis one of the most popular and sought-after device-based skincare procedures.

Chapter 3
Intense pulsed light (IPL)

Lasers do not have a universal application because they emit only at one wavelength. Yet, having a multifunctional device adapted to solve many problems would be highly beneficial!

Indeed, such devices exist and are based on intense pulsed light (IPL) technology. They emit in a wide range of wavelengths, and with the help of interchangeable light filters, it is possible to choose the wave (or waves) required in a particular case, or to use the entire generated spectrum (Gade A. et al., 2023).

Even though lasers also work with light radiation, IPL treatment "got" the prefix "photo" giving rise to the terms such as photoepilation and photorejuvenation. However, it is more accurate to call these technologies "procedures using sources of broadband optical radiation." This definition describes the essence of the method — emission in a wide range of wavelengths. In literature, another term denotes IPL: "flash-lamp, which reflects the pulsating nature of radiation," resulting in the generation of flashes of broadband light.

The main component of the IPL device is a quartz glass lamp filled with xenon gas with electrodes inside. The gas is ionized at the moment of the discharge between electrodes, and a light pulse comprising electromagnetic waves belonging to different parts of the spectrum is generated (**Fig. I-3-1**). Thus, IPL is characterized by so-called **polychromatic radiation** with wavelengths ranging from 400 to 1200 nm, extending from the visible light to the near-IR spectral range.

The second feature of IPL devices is **incoherence**. This means that the electromagnetic waves emitted by the lamp do not coincide with each other in phase and oscillate uncoordinated (apart), which renders the beam less focused.

Finally, IPL is **non-collimated**. Unlike a laser that produces a narrow light beam, IPL beam is divergent. This slightly reduces the intensity

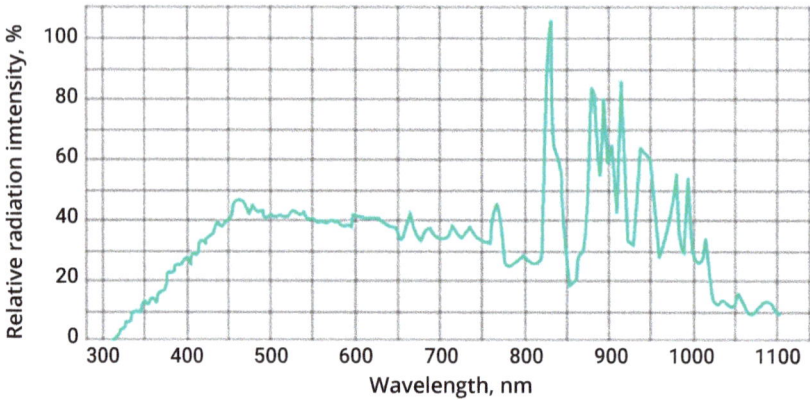

Figure I-3-1. Xenon flash lamp emission spectrum

of impact but expands the irradiation zone: a much larger area can be treated with one flash.

The principle of operation of IPL devices is based on selective photothermolysis, just as in the case of lasers. However, unlike lasers, which emit light of a single wavelength, IPL devices emit a wide range of wavelengths absorbed by different skin chromophores. This is both their advantage and disadvantage. On the one hand, IPL technology allows practitioners to target several significant chromophores simultaneously, thus solving many aesthetic problems with a single device. However, the downside is that the energy of the emitted light will be distributed among all these chromophores. The surface targets, such as pigment and dilated blood vessels, absorb most of the imparted energy. Higher energy parameters must therefore be used to heat deeper targets (these can be deep pigment and vascular defects, but also the collagen fibers in the dermis), which increases the risk of burns and other complications such as hyper- and hypopigmentation and scarring.

The history of IPL devices is linked to American physicians — phlebologist Mitchel P. Goldman and dermatologist Richard E. Fitzpatrick, who in 1990 described the use of high-intensity pulsed lamps as a tool for treating telangiectasias. In 1994, ESC Medical, now known as Lumenis, created the first IPL device, Photoderm. In 1995, it received

FDA approval as a device for treating telangiectasias on the lower extremities.

Modern IPL devices have undergone very significant technical changes: cooling systems and pulse splitting technology have appeared, and parameter setting has been improved and simplified. All this has made the IPL technology more comfortable and safer and has expanded the list of indications for its use.

The main features of IPL technologies, some of which can be interpreted as advantages or disadvantages depending on the circumstances, as presented below:

- Quick treatment of large areas
- Flashes may differ slightly from each other in energy and emission spectrum
- The large light spot size does not allow beam to focus on a point
- Direct contact of the tip with the skin
- Significant tip weight
- Gel application to cool and soften th skin during the treatment
- Multi-purpose use due to interchangeable light filters
- Low cost

The variation of individual flashes in energy and spectrum could be considered a shortcoming of the technology. Objectively speaking, however, it should be recognized that, although the flashes of light may be different, the differences observed are not so significant as to affect the procedure quality. Using a gel that partially cools and softens the skin can be seen as an advantage of the technology rather than a disadvantage. The transparent gel is designed to eliminate the air layer between the crystal and the skin and increases the epidermis's transparency by moisturizing it. However, according to some experts, the direct contact of the IPL tip with the skin is a disadvantage of this method. IPL technology uses a photoflash that is applied directly to the skin. In doing so, the light can affect collagen by dispersing along collagen fibers as light guides. At least, it is known that the structure of the collagen–elastin framework is markedly improved after IPL treatment (Knight J.M., Kautz G., 2019).

One of the important advantages of IPL devices is the long life of the emitter lamp (up to 70,000 pulses). Interchangeable light filters with optimal parameters (including different light spot sizes) are also highly beneficial, as they allow one device to solve various dermatological and esthetic problems.

With the same device, it is possible to affect blood-filled vessels (due to the absorption of light by hemoglobin), pigments in aging skin, spots, and unwanted hair, while its effects on water lead to changes in collagen, accompanied by the lifting and smoothing of fine lines and wrinkles, reduction of skin porosity, and thickening of skin tissue. It is important to note that lifting can be achieved by other means (high-intensity focused ultrasound [HIFU], radiofrequency [RF], thread lifting), but after these effects, the color and texture of the skin practically do not change. After IPL treatment, skin color and tone visibly improve, and this is one of the main advantages of IPL technologies (Husain Z., Alster T.S., 2016).

Chapter 4
Low-intensity laser therapy

As we have already mentioned, the marked effect of laser radiation on the chromophore and its impact on the target structure depend on the energy (J) of laser radiation and its power (W). Accordingly, in addition to high-intensity lasers, low-level laser (light) therapy (LLLT) is also used in cosmetology.

LLLT is used for **photobiomodulation** (also known as **photomodulation**). This term refers to the process of irradiating the skin with low doses of near-IR light (630–1000 nm) to modulate (stimulate or inhibit) the functional activity of cells to achieve a positive therapeutic effect (Avci P. et al., 2013a).

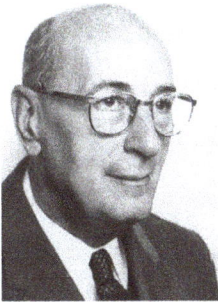

Endre Mester
(1903–1984)

The phenomenon of photobiostimulation was discovered in 1967 by Hungarian scientist Endre Mester (Semmelweis University Budapest, Hungary), who conducted experiments aiming to detect the carcinogenic effect of RUBY laser emitting red light with a wavelength of 694 nm. The scientist found no carcinogenic effect, but to his surprise he saw a distinct increase in hair growth on shaved areas exposed to radiation.

Further research on the phototherapeutic effect of LLLT mainly focused on the wound-healing potential. After the invention of light-emitting diodes (LEDs), which replaced bulky and expensive lasers, numerous compact photobiostimulation devices with various light pulses appeared on the market. The compactness and maneuverability of these light sources, their high efficiency in minimizing heat generation, and their use of a low-voltage power supply were considerable advantages over lasers, stimulating further research on photobiomodulation. Nowadays, these devices are actively conquering the market for home skincare devices.

The mechanism of LLLT action is still not precisely defined, but several assumptions have been made to explain the biophysical and physiological mechanisms underlying its effect on cells and tissues. Each assumption is based on a large body of experimental evidence (Hamblin M.R., 2016; Nestor M. et al., 2017).

While we will not detail all the hypotheses explaining the putative mechanisms of action of LLLT on biological tissues, we will list them briefly.

- **"Mitochondrial" hypothesis:** Red and IR light are absorbed by enzymes of the mitochondrial respiratory chain. This accelerates electron transport along the respiratory chain during oxidative phosphorylation, increasing the amount of adenosine triphosphate (ATP) in the cell and activating transcription factors.
- **The "oxidative stress" hypothesis:** Laser irradiation can cause three types of photochemical reactions: photo-oxidation of lipids in cell membranes, photoreactivation of the enzyme superoxide dismutase, and photolysis of nitric oxide (NO) complexes. These reactions result in the "release" of an increased amount of reactive oxygen species (ROS) and a state of "oxidative stress" in the cell, forcing it to mobilize its defense and detoxification systems.
- **"Copper" hypothesis:** Stimulation of wound healing by red light due to the activation of copper-containing tripeptide glycyl-L-histidyl-L-lysine (Cu:GHK) discovered by Loren Pickart in 1973. Cu:GHK is a powerful anti-inflammatory agent, limiting the degree of damage to tissue structures due to oxidative stress. It also serves as a signaling molecule that promotes tissue repair by activating the process of removing damaged proteins and replacing them with normal structural elements.
- **The "thermodynamic" hypothesis:** LLLT triggers physiological reactions due to the absorption of laser radiation by intracellular components (**Fig. I-4-1**; Moskvin S.V., 2021).

Numerous studies show anti-inflammatory, wound healing, stimulating, immunomodulating, lipolytic effects of LLLT. Accordingly, in dermatology and skincare, LLLT is used to treat inflammatory diseases (acne, atopic dermatitis, eczema, psoriasis, etc.), to accelerate healing

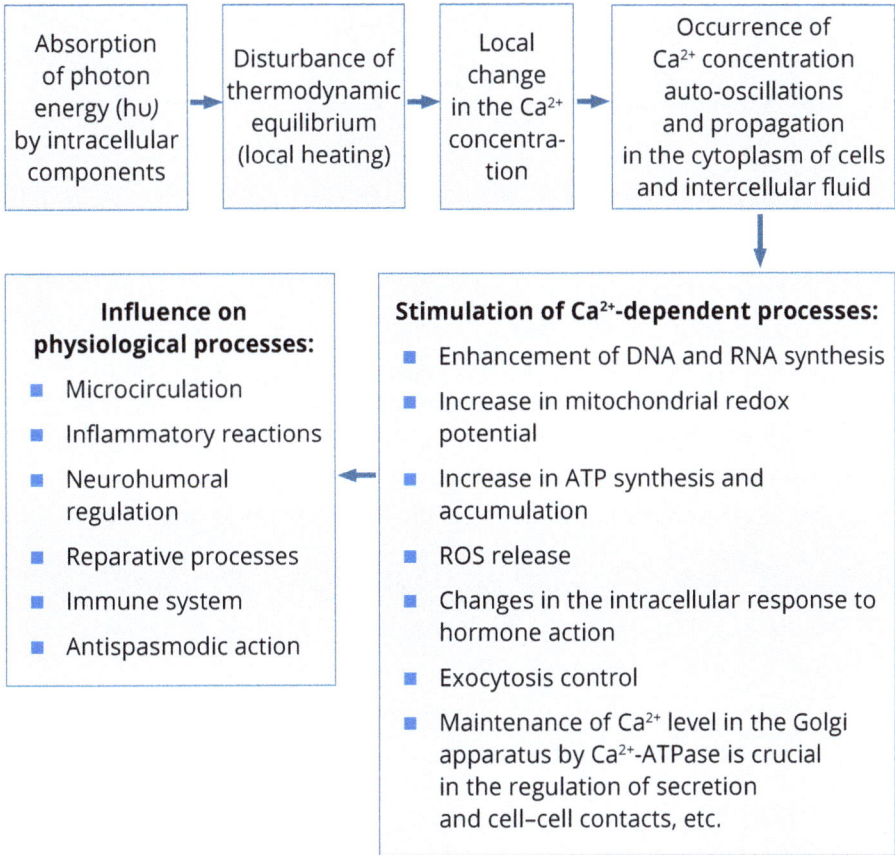

Figure I-4-1. Sequence of development of laser exposure-induced biological effects (according to Moskvin's thermodynamic hypothesis) (Moskvin S.V., 2021)

after aggressive procedures and normalize scar healing, to stimulate epidermal and dermal renewal, lipolysis and alopecia treatment, as well as for rejuvenation (Nestor M. et al., 2017; Couturaud V. et al., 2023).

Chapter 5
Photodynamic therapy

Photodynamic therapy (PDT) is a fast-growing minimally invasive treatment that was initially used in oncology. It is also based on selective photothermolysis, but rather than natural skin structures, the chromophores for irradiation are special compounds — photosensitizers and exogenous chromophores — administered externally. They are selected considering the ability of different cells to accumulate them (Rkein A.M., Ozog D.M., 2014).

Photosensitizers can be local or systemic. Only the former are used in cosmetic dermatology, as unlike systemic photosensitizers, they rarely cause delayed phototoxicity.

Three factors are necessary for the realization of PDT:
1. Photosensitizer
2. Light source
3. Oxygen

When photosensitizers absorb light, a photochemical reaction develops — molecular triplet oxygen is converted into singlet oxygen, and many highly active radicals are formed. Free radicals and singlet oxygen directly destroy target cells and damage microvessels (Castano A.P. et al., 2004).

Thus, **PDT is based on light absorption by a photosensitizer, which then produces reactive oxygen species (ROS), such as singlet oxygen, that destroy the structures that this photosensitizer accumulates**.

A variety of light sources, both laser and non-laser, can be utilized in PDT. The choice of source depends on the spectral characteristics of the photosensitizer used, as well as the localization and size of the target. Non-laser sources include xenon and mercury lamps. As for laser systems, these are dye lasers, solid-state lasers with double-frequency radiation, and IPL, but in recent years, Diode lasers have become the most popular and deservedly so.

In cosmetic dermatology, PDT is a new and rapidly developing method for treating inflammatory skin diseases such as acne, actinic keratosis, and psoriasis, as well as infectious skin diseases, including simple warts, acute condylomas, and cutaneous leishmaniasis. PDT is also used to treat signs of skin photoaging, and the range of indications for the application of this technology is constantly expanding (Darlenski R., Fluhr J.W., 2013; Lee C.N. et al., 2020).

Part II

Practical skills & clinical experience

Chapter 1
Laser rejuvenation

Age-related skin changes are characterized by the appearance of superficial and deep wrinkles, decreased elasticity and firmness, density reduction, formation of pigment and vascular defects, etc. Light technologies can help improve the skin condition in almost all these cases.

When we talk about laser rejuvenation procedures, we usually mean laser resurfacing and fractional ablative and non-ablative photothermolysis procedures, which we have already discussed above. Although removing age-related pigmentation and vascular defects also lead to "rejuvenation," we will discuss these technologies in detail in the following sections, and in this one, we will touch upon the variants of treatment in which the main chromophore is water.

1.1. How skin rejuvenation lasers work

Let's consider specific molecular mechanisms of such procedures using ablative CO_2 lasers, considered the "gold standard" of laser rejuvenation.

Biological reactions of the skin in response to CO_2 laser damage are both similar and qualitatively different from the healing of other types of wounds. Skin treatment with CO_2 laser is accompanied by the formation of thermal tissue damage — ablation, coagulation, and sublethal heat shock zones. The response to such damage is a well-organized and highly reproducible cascade that begins with a rapid increase in interleukin (IL-1β) and tumor necrosis factor-alpha (TNF-α) levels. These pro-inflammatory cytokines are involved in mechanisms related to the tissue repair process, and each induces the synthesis of matrix metalloproteinases (MMPs) required for the degradation and clearance of damaged dermal components (Heidari Beigvand H. et al., 2020).

1.1.1. Degradation reactions

Several MMP types are involved in the degradation of damaged collagen — the same types involved in age-related degradation of collagen fibers (Orringer J.S. et al., 2004).

Collagenase 1 (MMP-1) is responsible for the first step. Its level starts to increase three days after treatment, and after a week, it increases 40,000 times.

Seven days after exposure, another important collagen-destroying enzyme — gelatinase B (MMP-9) — and stromelysin (MMP-3) — an enzyme that destroys partially degraded collagen and other protein structures of the matrix (proteoglycans and elastin) — reach their peak values.

The MMP-1 and MMP-3 levels decrease sharply two weeks after the procedure, but the MMP-9 level decreases much more slowly. According to the available studies, MMP-9 levels remained almost at peak values (42 times higher than at the beginning) even 28 days after the procedure (**Fig. II-1-1**) (Orringer J.S. et al., 2004).

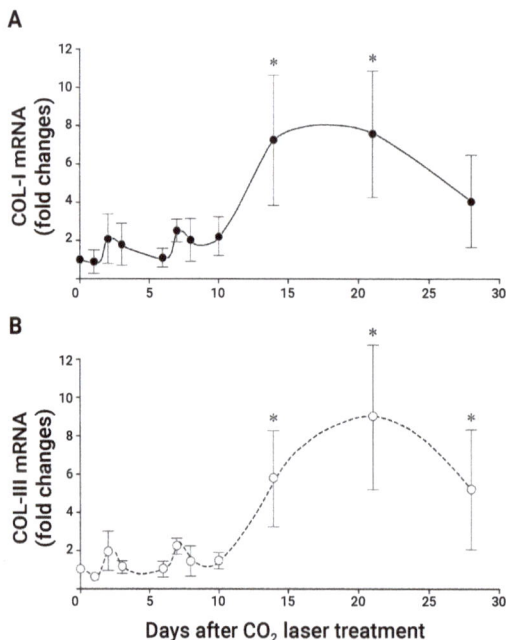

Figure II-1-1. Induction of (A) type I (COL-I) and (B) type III (COL-III) procollagen messenger RNA (mRNA) in human skin *in vivo* by carbon dioxide (CO_2) laser resurfacing (adapted from Orringer J.S. et al., 2004)

Skin samples were obtained at the indicated times after treatment. Type I procollagen and type III pro-collagen mRNA levels were quantified by reverse transcriptase–polymerase chain reaction. n = 4 to 11 at each time point; asterisk indicates P.05 *vs.* untreated control skin. Data points represent means; limit lines denote standard errors.

1.1.2. Reduction reactions

It is assumed that the cleavage of fragmented photodamaged collagen under the action of MMP is a stimulus for forming and depositing new collagen. The coincidence of these reactions in time confirms this assertion. Thus, on day 10 after CO_2 laser exposure, activation of type I and III procollagen synthesis was noted, which peaked between weeks 2 and 3 after treatment, when MMP-1 and MMP-3 levels had already decreased. For example, MMP-1 levels fall just before the bulk of new collagen accumulates, which protects collagen from degradation. In addition, new collagen formation supports increased levels of transforming growth factor-beta (TGF-β1), which has potent profibrotic properties. Its amount peaks two days after treatment and remains elevated for at least 28 days (**Fig. II-1-2**) (Orringer J.S. et al., 2004).

It has been observed that the level of collagenase 3 (MMP-13) increases later than MMP-1, MMP-3, and MMP-9, reaching a peak two weeks after CO_2 laser treatment. MMP-13 is thought to be involved in collagen remodeling.

This occurs at later stages of wound healing rather than at the initial stage of collagen degradation, supporting the concept that the work of

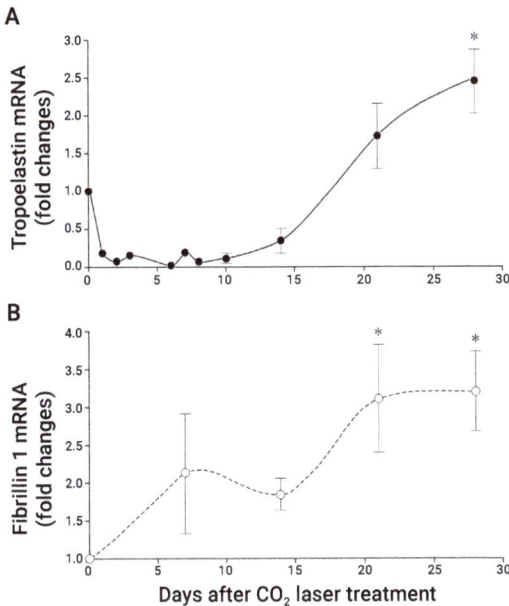

Figure II-1-2. Induction of (A) tropoelastin and (B) fibrillin 1 messenger RNA (mRNA) in human skin *in vivo* by CO_2 laser resurfacing (adapted from Orringer J.S. et al., 2004)

Skin samples were obtained at the indicated times after treatment. Tropoelastin and fibrillin 1 mRNA levels were quantified by reverse transcriptase–polymerase chain reaction. n = 4 at each time point; asterisk indicates P.05 *vs.* untreated control skin. Data points represent means; limit lines denote standard errors.

MMP-13 is directed toward remodeling newly formed collagen rather than destroying old collagen.

Studies show that procollagen type I and III levels remain elevated for at least six months after laser resurfacing. This is consistent with clinical observations — patients' skin improves for many months after laser resurfacing.

In addition to the increase in collagen after exposure to CO_2 laser, researchers have found relatively small but clear changes in the levels of tropoelastin and fibrillin 1 — two major components of elastin fibers. Their levels increased 28 days after treatment, and in some cases tropoelastin matrix ribonucleic acid (mRNA) levels remained elevated six months after treatment. In addition, disorganized elastic fibers, a sign of photodamaged skin, may be displaced deeper into the dermis after resurfacing. All these molecular changes are characteristic of both continuous laser resurfacing and fractional ablative CO_2 laser treatment.

Finally, a qualitative difference between tissue healing reactions after CO_2 laser treatment and other types of healing is the absence of myofibroblasts (α-smooth muscle actin-positive fibroblasts). Myofibroblasts are specialized, differentiated fibroblasts that differ from dermal fibroblasts in their expression of α-smooth muscle actin, increased ability to contract collagen fibrils, and increased formation of type I collagen. They are found in wounds caused by injuries such as burns or surgical incisions and are associated with wound contracture and scarring because of healing. This difference may be due to the relatively superficial and controlled nature of CO_2 laser-induced injuries (Orringer J.S. et al., 2004).

1.2. Features of ablative and non-ablative fractional rejuvenation

Currently, laser resurfacing is rarely used, and has been almost completely replaced by **ablative fractional photothermolysis**.

Sometimes fractionated photothermolysis is performed above the basal membrane. Still, ablative fractionated beam treatments are often used to deliver laser energy deeper than the basal membrane to affect the dermis. In this case, a high-energy microbeam vaporizes tissue to the penetration depth and — depending on the laser wavelength, pulse duration, and energy density — it creates a coagulation zone around the perimeter of the ablative column. The indisputable advantage of ablative fractional technologies realized with ablative fractional lasers is the possibility of creating ideal skin area reduction conditions. The ablative column is "empty" immediately after the procedure. All tissues in the laser beam's path have been vaporized. In this case, there is an instantaneous reduction of the skin area, as there are physiological conditions for this — an instant lifting effect. The perforation hole on the basal membrane created by the ablative laser beam with a diameter of up to 250 μm closes in 2–3 days, eliminating the possibility of scar formation and minimizing the risk of complications. Greater depth of fractional work (1.5 mm and more) is combined with a pronounced reduction in skin area and a short rehabilitation period. Compared to ablative resurfacing of the skin over the entire surface, ablative fractional procedures provide very rapid re-epithelialization with very limited adverse side effects (mild post-inflammatory erythema for three months or less), while reducing the patient's rehabilitation time to four days or less. The method is effective when applied repeatedly (the course typically involves 2–6 procedures).

The mechanisms of **non-ablative fractionation** will be similar, although since there is less initial damage and response, the results will also be less pronounced. Therefore, a greater number of treatments is usually required to achieve effects comparable to those yielded by ablative fractionation.

However, non-ablative procedures do not cause damage to the *stratum corneum*. They are accompanied by rapid recovery of the epidermis — a full recovery of the basal layer due to active proliferation and migration of stem cells into the damaged areas is noted as early as 24 hours after exposure. Full recovery of the epidermis is usually completed by the seventh day. At the same time, as in the case of ablative fractional photothermolysis, skin color and tone improvement is noted because the newly formed epidermal cells contain a uniform and adequate amount of melanin.

As for the dermis, its recovery is longer but faster than that following ablative laser treatment. On the seventh day, in the undamaged areas located under the MTZ, increased expression of type III collagen is observed, and the processes of dermal collagen framework restructuring take place for 2–3 months, which leads to a reduction in wrinkle depth and the number of enlarged pores.

Thus, non-ablative fractional rejuvenation procedures are also quite effective. Although they necessitate a greater number of sessions, they require virtually no rehabilitation and carry a very low risk of complications.

1.3. Treatment parameters

In addition to the above-described basic laser exposure parameters, other factors will also play a role, including the **number of passes** during continuous laser resurfacing. With each pass, progressively deeper layers are "removed" and the depth of residual thermal damage to tissues increases. In the case of CO_2 lasers, the depth is limited due to the formation of a coagulation zone. For Er:YAG laser, coagulation is minimal, as there is mainly tissue ablation, so the number of passes and, therefore, the depth of resurfacing is theoretically unlimited.

In the case of **fractional** laser machines, the following parameters must be additionally considered.

- **MTZ depth:** Depends on the energy of the microbeam generated by the laser. The higher the energy, the deeper the thermal damage.
- **MTZ diameter:** Depends on the energy of the microbeam. This parameter determines the speed of healing — the higher it is, the fewer intact skin areas between MTZs and the slower the healing process. According to some data, if the MTZ diameter is greater than 500 μm, these processes are slowed down so much that the healing time becomes comparable to that required after laser resurfacing.
- **MTZ density:** The total number of MTZs in each square centimeter formed in one pass is called MTZ density per pass, and the total number of MTZs in the entire procedure is called total MTZ density.
- **Coverage percentage:** The ratio of the lesion area to the undamaged areas which is directly related to the MTZ diameter and total MTZ density. The greater the percentage, the more pronounced the results, but also the longer the rehabilitation. On average, the coverage percentage is 20%.

There are various scanning modes, such as MTZ patterns, that allow the distance between MTZs and their total density to be adjusted, thus changing the percentage of coverage. Modern devices allow practitioners to modify these and other parameters depending on the patient's individual characteristics and needs.

Multiple passes can also be performed with fractional lasers, but each subsequent pass increases the risk of MTZ overlap and deformation and, therefore, the likelihood of thermal damage.

1.4. Laser equipment

Table II-1-1 lists the main types of lasers used for ablative and non-ablative skin rejuvenation, which can be operated in continuous or fractionated beam mode. However, their effects will vary greatly depending on the specific technical capabilities of the devices and the parameters used. Let's just say that the possibilities are impressive, but only if certified devices are used (Heidari Beigvand H. et al., 2020).

Table II-1-1. Laser and IPL devices for skin rejuvenation

DEVICE	WAVELENGTH (nm)
Ablative technologies	
CO_2 (pulsed)	10,600
Er:YAG (pulsed)	2940
Er:YSGG (pulsed)	2790
Non-ablative technologies	
PDL	585–595
QS Nd:YAG (nano- and picosecond pulsed)	1064
Nd:YAG (long-pulsed)	1320, 1440
Diode (long-pulsed)	1450
Er:glass (long-pulsed)	1410, 1540, 1550
Thulium (long-pulsed)	1927
IPL	560–1200

In general, ablative laser resurfacing is performed once, whereas laser rejuvenation may consist of six sessions of non-ablative fractional treatment.

1.5. Photorejuvenation

Rejuvenation by IPL is called photorejuvenation. Unlike lasers, IPL affects several chromophores simultaneously, while the effect on water will not be decisive (Sales A.F.C. et al., 2022).

Thus, there are two types of effects underlying the rejuvenating action of IPL:

1. Destruction of excess pigment and unwanted vascular formations according to the principle of selective photothermolysis. Since skin aging is characterized not only by changes in its relief (wrinkles) and thinning but also by uneven pigmentation and the appearance of telangiectasias, color equalization has a noticeable rejuvenating effect.
2. The effect on the dermis, particularly collagen, leads to wrinkle smoothing, enlarged pore narrowing, and increased skin turgor and elasticity. Although most of the IPL energy is "intercepted" by melanin and hemoglobin, it is assumed that this effect is realized by heating the deep layers of the skin with the long-wave parts of the IPL spectrum (closer to 1200 nm). In addition, it has been shown that skin fibroblast stimulation by long-wave radiation results in increased synthesis of extracellular matrix proteins. This causes at least partial restoration of skin thickness and is realized due to the stimulating effect of IPL on TGF-β and synthesis of new collagen type III.

Fine wrinkles respond better to IPL treatment than deep wrinkles, but several sessions are required to attain visible results. As a rule, obtaining a visible effect requires 3–6 sessions 3–4 weeks apart, but the exact number is determined individually. It is recommended that the course be repeated once a year (DiBernardo B.E., Pozner J.N., 2016).

Chapter 2
Removing skin tissue

Tissue ablation using CO_2 lasers is currently one of the most effective mechanisms for the removal of skin tissue, including benign pigmented lesions, papillomas, warts, seborrheic and actinic keratosis, xanthelasma, onychomycosis, etc. (Omi T., Numano K., 2014; Maranda E.L. et al., 2016; Wollina U., 2018; Zhang J. et al., 2018).

For the use of laser light as a surgical instrument (the so-called laser scalpel), the most important aspect is that the laser light beam is collimated, i.e., has a small divergence. This property of laser light gives the laser beam, in surgical terms, sharpness, resulting in a spot diameter of 0.1–0.3 mm. However, the main advantage of a laser scalpel compared to a conventional scalpel is that, in the process of dissection, vessels with a lumen of less than 0.5 mm are blocked. As a result, the dissection is almost bloodless. The depth of soft tissue dissection and blood-stopping (hemostatic) effect depends on the speed with which the laser beam is guided along the incision line and the laser beam radiation density in the spot (i.e., the power per 1 cm^2):

- Dissection: at 50–100 W/cm^2
- Vaporization: at 500–850 W/cm^2
- Coagulation: at 50–150 W/cm^2

It is important to note that the effect is determined only by the energy flux density and not by the type of laser.

With the help of lasers, it is possible to perform procedures at the level of a single cell, which is the fundamental spatial limit of laser surgery. Still, this limit has yet to be reached due to macro-level side effects from heat and shockwaves caused by the accompanying unwanted impacts on surrounding tissues. From a physics point of view, these effects can be avoided if the exposure time is shorter than the duration of heat energy exchange and shockwave propagation. To this end, an attempt was made to use lasers with light pulse duration in the picosecond (10^{-12} s) range (Amini-Nik S. et al., 2010). Such optimized exposure of tissues to light pulses should represent the most effective possible mechanism for cutting biological tissues with minimal induced damage. Indeed, Amini-Nik and colleagues (2010) have verified this using a comparative study of wound healing (linear incisions on the skin of mice) after exposure to a picosecond laser, surgical 2940-nm Er:YAG, and scalpel. First, the number of living cells in the same volume of skin biopsy from the wound, assessed by ATP content (luciferase test), was different. Namely, around the wound after scalpel incision and in the wound induced by Er:YAG laser, there were almost 50% as many live cells and 150% as many after picosecond laser. Two weeks later, the size of wounds from the picosecond laser was 50% smaller than those from the conventional surgical laser. About 50% weaker activation of β-catenin and TGF-β was also observed after picosecond laser exposure, indicating less damage to the extracellular matrix. Schematically, the effects of scalpel and conventional and picosecond lasers on the skin are shown in **Fig. II-2-1**.

In addition, 585–595-nm PDL and 532-nm potassium-titanyl-phosphate (KTP) laser can also be used to remove warts. PDL has been shown to destroy the vascular network supplying the warts, while 532-nm Nd:YAG radiation destroys melanin-containing cells.

The efficacy of 1064-nm Nd:YAG in **onychomycosis** is also being actively investigated. Back in 2010, the U.S. FDA approved the laser therapy for onychomycosis using long-pulsed 1064-nm Nd:YAG, but the mechanism of its specific action is still being studied. There is some evidence that exposure to Nd:YAG can inhibit the growth of *Trichophyton rubrum* fungi *in vitro*, but the available information on the ability of laser therapy to prevent or inhibit fungal growth is highly controversial. However, the success of laser therapy in onychomycosis depends mainly on the chosen exposure parameters. According to recent studies, it should be a long-term therapy (at least eight weeks), followed by a maintenance course, and the use of high irradiation energy parameters is advised.

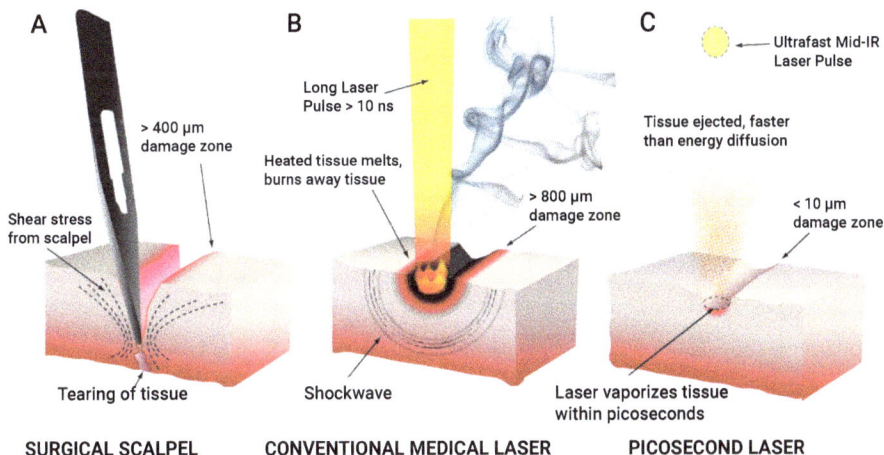

A
> 400 μm
damage zone

Shear stress
from scalpel

Tearing of tissue

SURGICAL SCALPEL

B
Long Laser
Pulse > 10 ns

Heated tissue melts,
burns away tissue

> 800 μm
damage zone

Shockwave

CONVENTIONAL MEDICAL LASER

C
Ultrafast Mid-IR
Laser Pulse

Tissue ejected, faster
than energy diffusion

< 10 μm
damage zone

Laser vaporizes tissue
within picoseconds

PICOSECOND LASER

Figure II-2-1. Schematic of cutting modalities

(A) The mechanical scalpel cuts skin by producing shear forces which exceed the elastic limit of the tissue. This causes a border of damage around the incision which reaches as far as 400 μm from the incision boundaries.

(B) Conventional surgical lasers cut by depositing heat until the tissue melts or burns away. The damage zone in this case can reach up to 800 μm away from the ablated edge.

(C) By contrast, the well-absorbed picosecond pulses cause the superheating of water inside the tissue on the picosecond timescale, ejecting the tissue faster than energy can diffuse to the surrounding area. The remaining adjacent tissue shows significantly less damage compared to the other two modalities (adapted from Amini-Nik S. et al., 2010).

Chapter 3
Vascular lesions

Vascular skin pathology is among the most common reasons for visiting aesthetic clinics, ranking third after hair removal and treatment for aging signs. This is due to three reasons:

1. Diversity of cutaneous vascular alterations
2. High frequency of occurrence
3. Proven high clinical effectiveness of laser technologies

The success of laser therapy in vascular lesions depends on various factors and, to a large extent, on the operator's skills. Physicians using vascular lasers must have the competence necessary to **correctly diagnose vascular skin lesions, explain the necessary nuances of treatment, assess the possible risks of therapy, select the parameters of laser exposure, and ensure safety during the procedure**.

3.1. Diagnosis

Vascular lesions can manifest as:

- **Vasodilation** (mainly capillary vasodilation), which leads to increased blood flow.
- **Capillary** constriction (vasoconstriction) and, consequently, a decrease in blood flow.
- **Violation of the vascular wall permeability**, which leads to impaired transport of substances from blood to tissues and vice versa, as well as to exudation of plasma and release of blood elements into dermal tissues (diapedesis).
- **Violation of vascular reactivity**, manifested by changes in mechanoreactivity (dermographism), thermoreactivity, neuro

reactivity, and hormonal reactivity, which may underlie the development of various pathological reactions to endogenous stimuli.

The localization of vascular lesions is very diverse in depth (**Table II-3-1**) and area — from limited foci (sometimes very small within one microcirculatory unit) to diffuse and even generalized, occupying significant areas or almost the entire skin.

Table II-3-1. Location of different types of skin vascular pathology

LEVEL	PATHOLOGY	DEPTH, µm
Subepidermal	• Superficial telangiectasias (TAE) in photoaging • Erythema in inflammatory skin diseases • Capillary angiodysplasia (CAD), also known as port-wine stain • Neovasculogenesis in scarring • Atrophodermia	40–50 70–260
Dermal	• Deep secondary TAE in severe photoaging • Age-related TAE • TAE in rosacea • TAE in collagenosis • Vasculitis • CAD • Cherry and spider angiomas	460–2235
Subdermal	• Venulectasias (blue reticular vessels 1–3 mm in diameter) • Angiomas and hemangiomas • Arteriovenous malformations • Venous malformations	1560–4000
Subcutaneous	• Hemangiomas • Arteriovenous malformations • Venous malformations • Reticular varicose • Saphenous veins pathologies	1800–4750 and deeper

It is essential to realize that correct diagnosis is the basis for successful therapy. A significant number of patients with vascular birthmarks receive ineffective and potentially dangerous treatment based on an incorrect diagnosis. To determine the exact nature of the vascular pathology, a detailed history and a thorough patient examination are necessary (Gloviczki P. et al., 2023).

According to the Grading of Recommendations, Assessment, Development and Evaluation (GRADE), most congenital and acquired vascular skin lesions belong to **class 1A** laser therapy. Class 1A recommendations are "strong" and have a meaningful evidence base. They should apply to most patients. Clinicians should only disregard these recommendations if a clear and convincing rationale exists for an alternative approach.

Currently, laser therapy can be used for the following vascular defects:

1. **Vascular malformations:**
   - Congenital vascular tumors (various forms of infantile hemangiomas, congenital hemangiomas, pyogenic granuloma, angiokeratoma)
   - Vascular malformations: port-wine stains — both as a separate pathology and associated with other anomalies (Sturge–Weber syndrome, Klippel–Trenaunay syndrome, etc.), telangiectasia (TAE), nevus simplex, venous malformations
2. **Acquired vascular lesions of the skin:**
   - Facial TAE
   - Rosacea
   - Spider angioma
   - Venous angioma
   - Cherry angioma
   - Senile angioma
   - Poikiloderma of Civatte
   - Pyogenic granuloma
   - Angiofibroma
   - Skin lesions in Kaposi's sarcoma
   - TAE of the lower extremities
   - Red and hypertrophic scars
   - Viral warts

- "Fresh" red stretch marks
- Inflammatory linear verrucous epidermal nevus
- Acne
- Psoriasis

Lasers are not recommended for treating arterial malformations because of the low evidence base (**class 1C**).

3.2. How do vascular lasers and IPL work

The target in treating vascular pathology is red blood cell hemoglobin, located in numerous dilated dermal vessels. Upon absorbing laser radiation, hemoglobin heats up and heats the vessel walls, which leads to their coagulation (photothermal effect) or rupture (photomechanical effect) (Zhang C. et al., 2023).

- **The photomechanical effect** manifests when a large amount of energy is transferred to the chromophore quickly. A so-called photodynamic shock occurs, the vessel ruptures and its contents are released into the tissue, leading to the formation of purpura, petechiae, and hemangiomas.
- **The photothermal effect** occurs with slower heating of the target (longer pulse) with gradual adhesion (coagulation) of the vessel. Blood, subjected to photocoagulation, forms a thermal coagulum — an amorphous accumulation of damaged and agglutinated erythrocytes and plasma components that clog the vascular lumen. Histologically, selective vessel damage with thrombosis, necrosis of the vessel wall, and perivascular collagen damage with relatively little thermal damage to the epidermis and dermis are noted.

Since IPL devices emit a broad range of wavelengths absorbed by different skin chromophores, most of this energy is absorbed by superficial targets such as pigment and dilated vessels. Higher energy parameters must be used to heat deeper targets, which increases the risk of burns and other complications, such as hyper- and hypopigmentation, and scarring (Sheptii O.V., 2018).

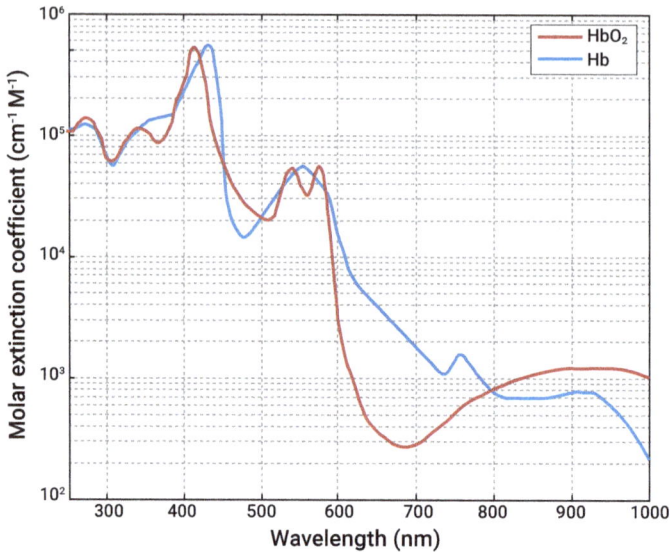

Figure II-3-1. Absorption curves of oxyhemoglobin (HbO_2) and deoxyhemoglobin (Hb)

3.3. Important parameters of vascular lasers

Wavelength

Regardless of the type of vascular lesions (arterial, venous, or capillary origin), hemoglobin remains the primary target for laser treatment (**Fig. II-3-1**):

- In small superficial vessels (mainly on the face and neck), the target is **oxyhemoglobin**, which has a maximum absorption peaks at 542 nm and 577 nm.
- In vessels on the legs, which are usually deeper and contain more **deoxyhemoglobin**, light of 800–1200 nm is used.
- In postcapillary venous malformations such as port-wine stains, 630–780-nm light is adopted.

The longer the wavelength, the deeper the radiation penetrates the skin (**Fig. II-3-2**). For example, Nd:YAG radiation of 1064 nm can penetrate several millimeters below the epidermis. **Longer wavelength light "bypasses" epidermal melanin, making it relatively safe for**

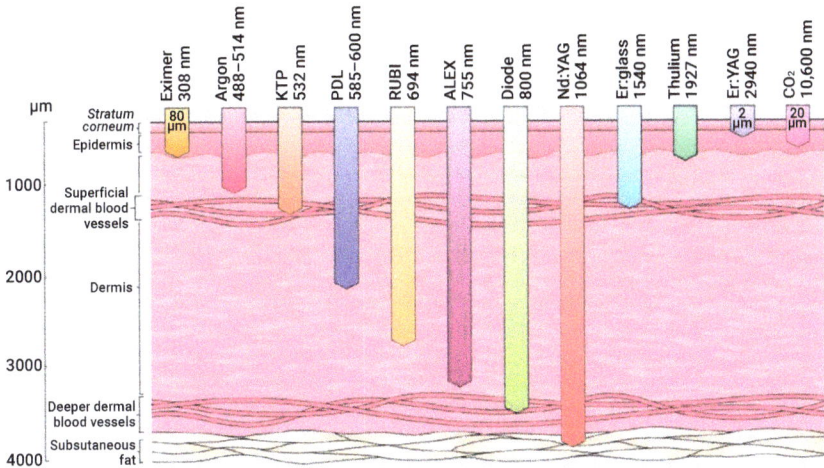

Figure II-3-2. Depth of penetration of laser radiation (Image adapted from Plastic Surgery Key)

darker skin types. However, coagulation of a deep vessel requires a much higher radiation energy density.

Infrared radiation treats deeper "blue" vessels more effectively, while shorter-wavelength light is more effective for superficial "red" telangiectasias.

Pulse duration

As noted previously, the effective and safe pulse duration for removing specific targets is determined based on the **thermal relaxation time (TRT)**. In vascular lesions, our target is not the hemoglobin itself but the vessel wall. According to the enhanced selective photothermolysis, hemoglobin is used as a target for heating with the expectation that the heat generated will be sufficient to damage the vascular wall. Therefore, pulse duration should be determined based on the blood flow volume and vessel diameter (**Table II-3-2**).

Table II-3-2. Thermal relaxation time of different skin structures

TARGET	SIZE, μm	TRT, ms
Melanosoma	0.1–0.5	0.25
Hair follicle	200	18
Vessels	50	1.2
	100	4.8
	200	19
	300	42.6
	400	160

For estimating the blood flow, the following parameters should be considered: the erythrocyte diameter is 7–10 μm, the average diameter of a capillary is 5–10 μm, and the blood flow velocity is 0.5–1 mm/s. Each blood particle is within the capillary for approximately one second. Thus, there may be only one erythrocyte in the lumen of malformed capillaries. As it moves slowly, its hemoglobin just transfers the energy that will lead to thermolysis of the vascular wall (coagulation or rupture depending on the pulse duration). Blood velocity in arterioles is 3 mm/s, while it is lower in venules — about 0.7 mm/s (due to lower pressure). Venules also have a significantly larger diameter than capillaries. In larger vessels, there are many red blood cells, and their speed is greater, so such vessels are much more difficult to remove. In this case, a different pulse duration should be used, and a large spot size may help.

Pulse frequency

Overlapping pulses or high pulse rates can result in thermal damage to tissue. However, in certain situations and in the hands of an experienced practitioner, this technique can yield good results — accumulated pulses with lower energy density can produce effects like a single higher-energy density pulse (IPL) on the target. For example, treating superficial facial TEA using the "pulse accumulation" technique can improve clinical outcomes without significantly increasing the risk of adverse side effects.

Spot size

Blood is in continuous motion. Accordingly, we are dealing with a dynamic chromophore. A new portion of blood "takes up" the heat generated by the absorption of laser energy, protecting the vessel from overheating. Therefore, a larger spot size is recommended to increase the circulating blood heating rate. In addition, a larger spot size promotes deeper penetration of laser light into the skin at equal radiation parameters.

Cooling

We must deliver high-energy pulses to targets deep in the skin to treat vascular lesions while minimizing damage to keratinocytes and melanocytes. This is mainly achieved by cooling the epidermis using a cryogenic spray, chilled air jet, or sapphire contact tips.

It must be remembered that remote cooling devices rapidly reduce epidermal temperature without affecting the chromophore. However, when contact cooling is used, the pressure on the skin and the low sapphire temperatures may reduce hemoglobin's desired absorption of laser energy.

3.4. Vascular lasers

Table II-3-3 summarizes the main types of devices currently used to treat various vascular lesions (Giovanni C. et al., 2023).

Table II-3-3. Vascular lasers and IPL

DEVICE	TARGETS / DEPTH	INDICATIONS	DISADVANTAGES
KTP 532 nm (green)	Oxyhemoglobin > melanin; 1 mm	• Facial TAE • Diffuse erythema • Rosacea • Cherry and spider angiomas • Poikiloderma of Civatte • Port-wine stains • TAE on legs (< 1 mm)	Usually used for more superficial vessels and epidermal damage in dark-skinned people (dyschromia and textural changes, sometimes scarring)
PDL 585, 595 nm (yellow)	Oxyhemoglobin > melanin; 1–1.5 mm	• Port-wine stains • Infantile hemangioma • TAE on the face • Rosacea • Cherry and spider angioma • Poikiloderma of Civatte • TAE on the legs	Pain, purpura (especially with a short-pulsed mode and high energy density); mainly used for more superficial vessels
ALEX 755 nm (infrared)	Melanin > deoxyhemoglobin > hemoglobin; 2–3 mm	• Port-wine stains • TAE on legs (< 2 mm)	High risk of hyperpigmentation and scarring, especially in dark phototypes

Continued on p. 72

DEVICE	TARGETS / DEPTH	INDICATIONS	DISADVANTAGES
Diode laser 800–983 nm (infrared)	Oxyhemoglobin ≥ melanin Above 900 nm low melanin absorption; 3–5 mm	• Facial TAE • Port-wine stains • Venous pooling • TAE on the legs	More suitable for large vessels; not enough clinical data on efficacy so far
Nd:YAG 1064 nm (infrared)	The melanin-to-blood absorption ratio is similar to PDL, but higher energy is required due to lower absorption; 5–6 mm	• Port-wine stains • Infantile hemangioma • TAE and venous ectasis of the lower extremities • Venous malformations • Pyogenic granuloma • Venous pooling	Painful, risk of deep damage and scarring
IPL 500–1200 nm	Filters for vascular lesions (550 and 570 nm, i.e., mainly yellow and red light)	• Facial TAE • Diffuse erythema • Rosacea • Port-wine stains • Thin TAE on legs • Poikiloderma of Civatte	Pain, heat burns, dyspigmentation; difficult to establish reliable treatment parameters due to technical differences across devices

3.5. Factors influencing the clinical results

The main factors affecting the efficacy and safety of laser therapy for vascular abnormalities are summarized below.

Dark phototype IV–V and tanned skin
Problem

Competitive light absorption by melanin worsens its interaction with oxyhemoglobin, increasing the risk of burns, scarring, hypopigmentation, and post-inflammatory hyperpigmentation.

Decision
- Use of 585–600-nm lasers in long-pulsed mode.

- Use of IR (800–1064 nm) lasers due to low absorption by melanin.
- The general recommendation for the client is to avoid sunlight for one month before the treatment and at least one month after, and to use sunscreens. However, the attending physician should individually determine the specific sun protection options and duration.

Vascular depth
Problem
Superficial TAEs can be treated faster and more easily with IPL, KTP, and PDL devices. Deep TAEs have a larger caliber, which requires a long-pulsed mode, high energy density, large spot size, and longer wavelengths.

Decision
Combining different devices, e.g., PDL/Nd:YAG or IPL/Nd:YAG, is preferable.

Blood flow velocity
Problem
For low-flow vessels (capillary angiodysplasia [CAD], venous and lymphatic malformations), coagulation becomes easier and faster. For high-flow vessels (centrofacial TAE, lower extremities, arteriovenous/arterial malformations), vessel recanalization can occur.

Decision
- Use of PDL or IPL with high energy density
- Use of 800–1064-nm lasers for maximal heating of the vessel intima
- Several sessions
- Combined protocols

Biophysical factors
Problem
When light hits the skin, the following biophysical processes occur:
- **Reflection:** About 5–7% of light is reflected at the *stratum corneum*. Increased reflection is due to poor skin contact.

- **Scattering:** This is mainly due to dermal collagen. Scattering is important because it rapidly reduces the energy flux density for the target chromophore.
- **Competitive absorption:** Oxyhemoglobin competes with melanin in the visible part of the spectrum (Ying Z.X. et al., 2020).

Decision
- Minimizing reflection: good fit to the skin and use of contact medium (transparent gel in IPL and KTP treatments).
- Minimizing scattering: scattering decreases with increasing wavelength, making longer wavelengths ideal for delivering energy to deep skin layers.
- Eliminating competitive absorption: the treatment should start with pigment removal, followed by blood vessels. In addition, in excessive keratinization, the skin should be well-cleaned and exfoliated by superficial chemical peeling.

Equipment
Problem
Use of low-quality equipment is associated with risks of complications, lack of results, and the inability to predict them.

Decision
Selection of certified equipment from well-known brands.

Patient responsibility
Problem
Ignoring the doctor's recommendations (visiting the bath, sauna, gym, taking part in a physical activity that increases blood circulation in the treatment area, alcohol consumption, insolation) contributes to vessel recanalization.

Decision
Clear recommendations, mandating that the patient signs informed consent. Denial of treatment to inadequate patients.

3.6. Practical recommendations

Vascular lasers generate high-energy radiation. Thus, their improper use, inadequate preparation for the procedure, and suboptimal post-procedure management of patients can cause serious side effects. Photographing the patient before, during, and after the treatment is highly recommended to evaluate the results and resolve disputes. Adherence to the recommendations outlined below will help improve the procedure effectiveness and safety.

3.6.1. Before the session

After diagnosing a vascular skin lesion, but before laser therapy, it is necessary to obtain answers to the questions listed below.

- Has the patient previously received any treatment that may attenuate the effect of the vascular laser (for example, electrocoagulation or other manipulations such as laser or IPL that provoke fibrosis in the area of exposure)? Fibrosis can also occur in the case of sclerotherapy or intralesional injection of corticosteroids in treating hemangiomas.
- Has the patient experienced any side effects or complications characterized as vascular pathology?
- Have there been episodes of post-inflammatory hyperpigmentation and excessive scarring?
- What is the patient's phototype?

In addition, it is essential to set realistic expectations for the patient. Patients with TAEs should be ready for 1–3 sessions, those with rosacea will require up to 4–5 sessions, and for the greatest effect in treating port-wine stains, the sessions can be stretched to two years.

Before the procedure, the patient must sign an informed consent form, which will explain the side effects and possible complications of laser treatment, as well as methods for their prevention and mitigation.

3.6.2. Basic principles of laser treatment

In general, the following principles should be adhered to in laser treatment of vascular lesions:

- Small vessels — shorter pulses
- Large vessels — longer pulses
- Deeper vessels — larger spot size, longer wavelength, and longer pulse duration combined with cooling to protect the epidermis
- Darker phototypes — longer wavelength, longer pulse duration and intervals

The treatment area should be thoroughly cleaned of makeup. Even though laser treatment of vascular lesions is a painful procedure, most patients do not need anesthesia.

The procedure should start with **test parameters**, using a suitable pulse duration, spot size, and optimal energy density (the maximum allowed for the clinical case).

When treating areas prone to scarring (chest and neck) and areas with sensitive and thin skin (periorbital area), a **10–20% reduction in energy** is required. In addition, to minimize scarring, the percentage of pulse overlap should not exceed 10%. Reduction in laser energy in the area of bony protrusions that reflect the laser beam is also recommended.

Most vascular lesions require more than one treatment session with 2–6 week or longer intervals between treatments for optimal healing. Shortening the intervals may induce fibrosis, impairing laser penetration.

3.6.3. Post-session care

The recovery period after the session typically lasts 7–10 days. Care on the first day includes applying cold presses in the treatment area (e.g., an ice pack wrapped in a napkin) for 10–15 minutes at 4-hour intervals. If the treatment is performed in the eye area or on the cheeks, sleeping on the back with the head elevated is recommended.

The laser-treated area is extremely sensitive. Thus, any skin treatment in the first 7–10 days must be done carefully. Patients should also be advised not to traumatize or scratch the treated area. A mild, non-irritating soap can be used to clean the treated areas twice a day. Bepanten cream provides the moisturizing required, while accelerating healing. Vaseline-based ointments (Aquaphor, Bepanten ointment, methyluracil) can be used to treat blisters.

Makeup can be applied after treatment unless swelling is present or blisters form. While the skin is healing, the patient should avoid swimming in a pool or playing sports. Bathing is allowed, but prolonged soaking or sauna use is not recommended.

To prevent post-inflammatory hyperpigmentation, sunscreen with 50+ sun protection factor (SPF) is recommended for the entire course of treatment, including at least four weeks before and after the intervention. The treating physician should determine the options and duration of sun protection.

The response to treatment is not evaluated immediately after the skin healing process. For example, the results of leg vein treatment can be seen 2–3 months after the procedure.

3.6.4. Adverse events and complications

Since laser therapy utilizes high levels of energy, procedures are often accompanied by side effects and complications. Some are unavoidable, while the risk of developing others can be reduced. Let's take a look at the most common ones.

- **Pain** can signal possible adverse reactions during the procedure, so anesthesia should be avoided if possible.
- **Purpura and hematomas** form immediately after laser treatment in cases of "fragile" vessel exposure to aggressive modes. They disappear within 7–10 days.
- **Erythema and edema** occur a few minutes after laser treatment, most often when vascular defects under the eyes or on the neck are removed. They disappear within 3–5 days. Cooling during and immediately after the procedure reduces the severity of edema.
- **Discoloration, blisters, or crusts** rarely develop (mainly when high energies are used). Epidermal discoloration to gray or pale pallor — an early sign of skin damage indicating

the use of high energy densities — is observed for a few seconds. Blister formation, epidermal damage, and epidermal necrosis (in severe cases, dermal necrosis) occur later. The solution to the problem is intensive cooling, decreasing the energy density, and lengthening the pulse. Resolution of the resulting damage takes 1–2 weeks. To prevent the development of this complication, a test pulse should be applied 5 min before the start of the main protocol and the resulting spot should be evaluated.

- **Infection** is possible, but should resolve with local antiseptics or systemic antibiotics. It should be suspected when prolonged swelling, redness, crusting, pain, and increased local temperature is present.

- **Reactivation of *herpes simplex*** on the face (when removing a vascular defect on the facial skin) or genitals (when performing procedures on the legs). Prophylactically prescribed virostatic therapy (acyclovir, valacyclovir) if the patient has frequent recurrences of herpes infection (more than six per year) is recommended in these cases.

- **Hyperpigmentation** is more common in patients with darker skin types. The risk of its appearance increases with insolation. Post-procedural hyperpigmentation gradually disappears within 2–6 months. Bleaching cream can be applied to accelerate the process.

- **Hypopigmentation** occurs mainly when "excessive" laser parameters are used. Repigmentation usually takes 3–6 months. However, hypopigmentation can be permanent, especially on the neck, legs, and chest.

- **Skin texture changes** are mainly caused by over-treatment (high energy density) or overlapping patches.

- **Scarring** occurs for the same reasons as the previously discussed complication. Scarring after PDL and KTP treatments is rare, and is more likely after ALEX and Nd:YAG laser use due to the deeper energy penetration.

- **Therapy-resistant lesions** — some vascular lesions do not disappear completely despite best efforts.

3.7. Device of choice for different vascular lesions

Infantile hemangioma

Most infantile hemangiomas do not require treatment — 50% are completely resolved by age five, and 70% by age seven. Laser treatment of infantile hemangiomas remains controversial and should only be performed by experienced specialist with extensive knowledge of vascular anomalies. The use of vascular lasers is recommended as standalone therapy or in combination with other treatments (e.g., beta-blocker treatment + lasers for superficial infantile hemangiomas) when there are contraindications for systemic propranolol therapy, parental refusal of propranolol, or risk of significant side effects.

- PDL (595 nm), KTP (532 nm), and IPL may be used to treat superficial infantile hemangiomas.
- For deep thick infantile hemangiomas, Nd:YAG (1064 nm) or PDL/ Nd:YAG combination is recommended.

Although laser treatment of infantile hemangiomas should be performed early, in the initial stages of hemangioma formation, it is often difficult to predict whether the hemangioma will consist of only a superficial component or whether a deeper component will emerge later (which can occur despite successful treatment of the superficial component).

Capillary angiodysplasia

Unlike hemangiomas, capillary angiodysplasias (CAD, port-wine stains) never regress on their own. Therefore, **the earlier treatment is started, the more effective it is**.

- PDL (the greatest aesthetic effect), KTP, Nd:YAG, and IPL are used to treat CAD.

In most patients, significant spot lightening can be achieved, but not complete removal. For example, CAD located in the centrofacial area (upper lip, medial cheek area) or on the skin of the distal extremities cannot be removed entirely. Only 25% of lesions are completely removed after several treatments, whereby:

- Pink or red spots respond better to treatment than purple spots
- Spots on the face and neck respond better to treatment than those on the extremities
- The lateral parts of the face and forehead respond better to treatment than the centrofacial part

Some port-wine stains may reappear after treatment. Accordingly, follow-up photographs should be taken during treatment to evaluate its effectiveness and adjust the protocol.

For hypertrophic and resistant forms, ALEX, Diode, or Nd:YAG laser, as well as PDL with a longer pulse duration (1.5 to 10 ms) and a larger spot size, can be used.

Telangiectasias
- TAE on the face: PDL (595 nm), KTP (532 nm), and IPL. Clearing efficacy: at least 60–90% after 1–3 sessions.
- Deep "blue" TAE: long-wavelength lasers such as ALEX (755 nm), Diode (900 nm), or Nd:YAG (1064 nm). These devices carry a higher risk of side effects and complications.

Epidermal cooling reduces the risk of thermal damage and discomfort during the procedure. Cooling is particularly important when using short-wavelength lasers (KTP, PDL).

Telangiectasias and venulectasias (phlebectasias) of the lower extremities
The following laser therapy options are available for the treatment of superficial TAE of the lower extremities:
- Monotherapy of superficial aesthetic lesions is recommended in a superficial network of dilated small vessels (less than 1 mm in diameter) without signs of venous insufficiency or increased hydrostatic pressure typical for younger patients.
- Combined therapy (sclerotherapy/laser) yields the best results in the presence of dilated vessels of large caliber (1 mm or more).

Table II-3-4 summarizes the key treatment recommendations for different types of lower-extremity TAE.

Without normalizing hydrostatic pressure, successfully removing TAE on the lower extremities affected by of varicose veins is impossible.

Table II-3-4. Laser therapy for TAE on lower extremities

TAE	LASER TYPES AND OPTIMAL EXPOSURE PARAMETERS	DISADVANTAGES
Diameter: 0.1–1.0 mm Location: superficial, in the upper layers of the dermis (at the 300 and 1000 µm depth) Color: pink/red Main chromophore: oxyhemoglobin	PDL (595 nm) with variable pulse lengths (from 0.45 to 40 ms) Penetration depth: up to 1500 µm Optimal parameters: • spot: 7/10/3×10 mm • pulse duration: 10–30 ms • energy density: 6–20 J/cm²	High melanin absorption — high risk of pigmentation disorder
Diameter: 0.5–1.0 mm (optimum) Location: dermis/ hypodermis (1000–2000 µm depth range) Color: dark red/purple Main chromophores: oxyhemoglobin / deoxyhemoglobin	ALEX (755 nm) / Diode (800–1000 nm). Penetration depth: 2300–3000 µm Optimal parameters: • spot: 3–8 mm • pulse duration: 5–20 ms • energy density: 20–80 J/cm² depending on spot size	Temporary hyper-pigmentation may occur in patients with dark photo-type
Diameter: 1–5 mm Location: deep skin layers / hypodermis (up to 3000 µm) Color: magenta/blue Main chromophores: deoxyhemoglobin	Neodymium Nd:YAG: 1064 nm Penetration depth: up to 5000 µm Optimal parameters: • spot: 3–8 mm • pulse duration: 20–60 ms • energy density: 70–600 J/cm²	Pain/risk of skin damage — scarring, atrophy This laser allows the treatment of patients with dark skin phototypes (low absorption of radiation by melanin)

Poikiloderma of Civatte

This condition is caused by chronic over-insolation, so mandatory use of sunscreen is recommended.

- PDL (595 nm), KTP (532 nm), and IPL are effective for treating the poikiloderma of Civatte. In some cases, 2–3 sessions are required. In areas prone to scarring (neck, chest), it is recommended to reduce energy by 20–30%, use a large spot size (10 mm for PDL), and avoid overlapping pulses.
- Fractional ablation should be used to eliminate dyschromia, pigmentation, and skin texture changes.

3.8. Rosacea

Rosacea is a chronic polyetiological progressive facial dermatosis based on angioneurotic disorders, which we consider under vascular pathology.

In 2002, a **classification of rosacea** that includes four subtypes was developed:

- **Subtype I, or erythematoteleangiectatic rosacea:** defined by the presence of flushing in the central part of the face
- **Subtype II, or papulopustular rosacea:** the presence of persistent erythema and periodic rashes in the form of papules and pustules, with a centrilobular distribution
- **Subtype III, or phymatous rosacea:** characterized by thickened skin with irregular contours, affecting the ears, cheeks, chin (gnathophyma), forehead (metophyma), and nose (rhinophyma)
- **Subtype IV, or ophtalmorosacea:** lacrimation, burning, dry, itchy, and light-sensitive eyes combined with hyperemia

This classification is still considered vital in clinical practice, although it has undergone some refinements (van Zuuren E.J. et al., 2021).

3.8.1. Treatment strategy

The variety of etiologic and pathologic factors underlying dermatosis, its stage, and clinical picture determine which of the numerous ways will be used to treat rosacea. At present, there is an extensive arsenal of drug therapy modes, including those with anti-inflammatory, antihistamine, sedative, immunoprotective, and radioprotective action.

Phototherapy is currently considered the fastest and most effective way to treat rosacea. Laser light sources and IPL systems are used for this purpose (see **Table II-3-5**, **Fig. II-3-3**). Depending on the clinical manifestations, two directions in phototherapy for this disease can be distinguished:

1. Treatment of vascular and inflammatory changes in the skin
2. Treatment of dystrophic changes in tissues

Table II-3-5. Laser application depending on the clinical manifestation of rosacea

	DEVICE	EXPECTED RESULT
Vascular changes	• PDL (585, 595 nm) • IPL (500–1200 nm) • KTP (532, 540 nm) • Nd:YAG (1064 nm)	Reduction in the severity of clinical symptoms, complete removal of TAE and erythema
Inflammatory changes	• PDL (585, 595 nm) • KTP (532, 540 nm)	Reduction in the number of rashes, rapid remission achievement and maintenance
Deformational, hypertrophic tissue changes	• CO_2 (10,600 nm) • Er:YAG (2900 nm) • Nd:YAG (1064 nm)	Reduction of deformed tissue
Dystrophic changes in tissue structure	**Ablative fractional lasers** • CO_2 (10,600 nm) • Er:YAG (2940 nm) • Er:YAG + SMA (2940 nm) **Non-ablative fractional lasers** • Diode and Neodymium lasers (1440 nm) • Thulium laser (1927 nm) • Erbium laser (1550 nm)	Reduction in the severity of clinical symptoms, attainment of long-term remission

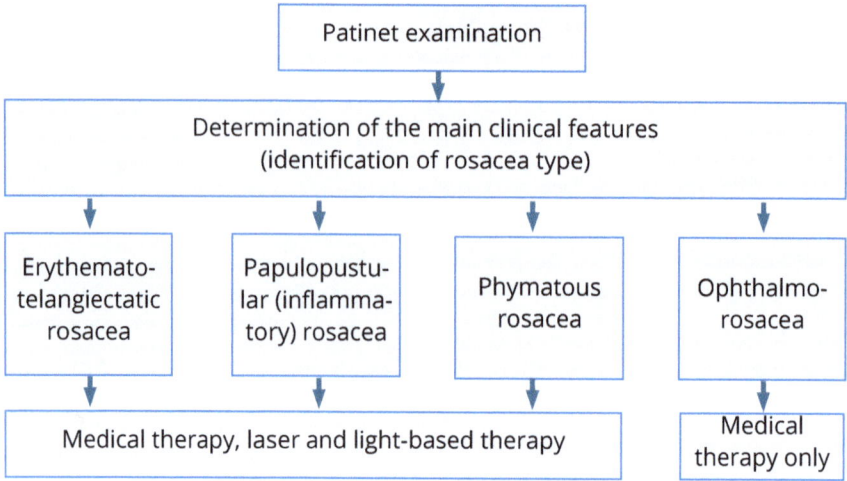

Figure II-3-3. Selecting treatment strategies for patients depending on the rosacea subtype

The aim of light-based therapy (phototherapy) for rosacea is to selectively remove pathological vessels without damaging the integrity of the skin and to achieve positive long-term results.

3.8.2. Vascular lesions

Several varieties of laser and IPL systems are currently used to treat vascular lesions (Zhang Y. et al., 2020).

Pulsed dye laser (PDL)

PDL wavelengths (577, 585, and 595 nm) coincide with the absorption peak of hemoglobin and thus affect the superficial vasculature. At the same time, they are not effective enough to remove deep vessels.

Studies conducted with PDL indicate a favorable effect of radiation at these wavelengths on erythema and telangiectasias, as well as a reduction in the number of rashes in the papulopustular type of rosacea. In addition, it is indicated that three months after the end of the treatment course, the level of neuropeptides involved in the microvascular pathophysiologic reaction is statistically significantly reduced, contributing to a decrease in the inflammatory response in the skin.

Previously, classical PDL led to the occurrence of purpura and dyschromia after treatment, but these issues have now been minimized by increasing the pulse duration.

Potassium-titanium-phosphate laser (KTP)

KTP (532 and 540 nm) removes linear and branching telangiectasias at various depths. Green light is in the absorption spectrum of hemoglobin, which allows a significant portion of the energy to be directed to coagulate vessels of various diameters.

It yields positive results in the treatment of erythema, telangiectasias, as well as papulopustular elements in the facial area. There is evidence in the literature of a decrease in the severity of the inflammatory response in the skin after KTP laser therapy.

Undesirable phenomena are insignificant (in the form of soreness, purpura, and hyperpigmentation) and are usually transient in nature. The disadvantage of the method is that radiation at these wavelengths interacts not only with hemoglobin, but also with melanin (albeit to a lesser extent), which increases the risk of post-inflammatory hyperpigmentation.

Neodymium laser (Nd:YAG)

Nd:YAG (1064 nm) has a positive effect on large and deep vessels. Since it is a long-pulsed laser, it is not commonly used to treat pathologically altered vessels in the face, as there is a high risk of complications, such as scarring and dyschromia. Nd:YAG is often utilized to remove vessels in the lower extremities.

Some literature sources indicate positive rosacea treatment outcomes with a long-pulsed ALEX/Nd:YAG dual-wavelength laser (755/1064 nm). The disadvantages are the presence of purpura and soreness, which are also transient in nature.

Intense pulsed light (IPL)

IPL systems (500–1200 nm) allow the removal of both superficial and deep vessels, which reduces the severity of erythema and telangiectasias. However, this method requires highly specialized clinical knowledge and practical experience to customize the procedure properly and reduce the risk of complications. The higher risk of complications is due to the active effect on many chromophores in the skin (melanin, hemoglobin, protein, water).

In 75–100% of patients in the early stages of rosacea, IPL treatments have an effect after one or two sessions, with few complications, such as purpura, scarring, and post-inflammatory hyperpigmentation.

3.8.3. Skin hypertrophy

Rhinophyma is a severe late complication of rosacea characterized by progressive hyperplasia of the sebaceous glands and connective tissue with involvement of the lower two-thirds of the nose.

Rosacea treatment is usually conservative and can only control the course of the disease. Now, drugs can reduce the severity of erythematous-telangiectatic, papular, and ocular manifestations, but there is no convincing evidence that medications can cause regression of rhinophyma. In this case, invasive techniques remain the best option for therapy aimed at deformed tissues.

Dissection of deformed tissue can be performed with the following types of lasers emitting in the IR range:

- CO_2 (10,600 nm)
- Er:YAG (2900 nm)
- Nd:YAG (1064 nm)

Infrared lasers provide an effective and targeted thermal impact on the lesions, guaranteeing optimal re-epithelialization. This makes them suitable for surgical interventions with a limited inflammatory response and promotes better tissue healing.

Unlike Er-based lasers, CO_2 lasers induce the most traumatic changes in tissues, but they can also provide a dry wound surface during surgery. The neodymium emitter can also ensure complete vessel coagulation and a "dry surgical field," which undoubtedly contributes to a favorable aesthetic effect. Still, its cutting properties are inferior to those of CO_2 lasers.

Ablative laser therapy can be used to equalize the shape of a deformed nose by partial excision of excess tissue structures. Despite transient edema, erythema, crusting, and the risk of dyspigmentation and scarring, the outcome can be aesthetically and psychologically acceptable.

Rhinophyma causes pronounced psychological and physiological problems in patients, but there is no ideal solution. The literature provides data on combined therapy in the form of surgical cytoreduction and fractional photothermolysis, which minimizes the risks of complications and yields better short- and long-term results.

3.8.4. Skin dystrophy

Ablative and non-ablative fractional lasers are used to remodel tissue structures.

It should be remembered that **light-based therapy for skin remodeling should be carried out only when the activity of the inflammatory response is completely reduced since the altered tissue structures are very sensitive to various stimuli, and symptom exacerbation is likely**.

In rosacea, it is reasonable to use a combined approach consisting of sequential solutions to various problems with the help of medication and laser/light-based therapy. Since the vascular component is the leading cause of the disease, using light-based technologies to destroy dilated vessels and control inflammatory processes is recommended. The use of laser light to correct connective tissue changes in the skin will lead to a significant improvement in the patient's appearance.

More information on the treatment and control of rosacea is provided in the *Rosacea and Couperosis in Cosmetic Dermatology & Skincare Practice* book.

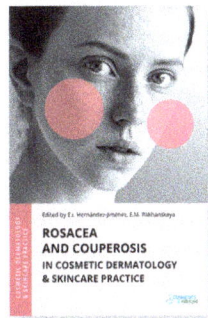

Edited by E.I. Hernández-Jiménez, E.M. Makhardova

ROSACEA
AND COUPEROSIS
IN COSMETIC DERMATOLOGY
& SKINCARE PRACTICE

Chapter 4
Pigmentary disorders

The appearance of pigmentary defects is associated with changes in the basic amount and distribution of melanin. Melanin is a pigment produced by melanocytes, large outgrowth cells localized in the basal layer of the epidermis. It is located in special vesicles surrounded by a membrane — melanosomes. As the pigment matures, these vesicles move to the periphery of the cells, enter the outgrowths of melanocytes, are transported to the surrounding basal keratinocytes, and, together with them, ascend to the more superficial layers of the epidermis (**Fig. II-4-1**).

Pigmentary disorders (dyschromias) fall into two broad groups:

- **Hyperpigmentation** (hypermelanosis, melanoderma) — an increase in melanin in the epidermis or dermis (Ko D. et al., 2023; Wang R.F. et al., 2023)
- **Hypopigmentation** (hypomelanosis, leukoderma) — a reduction or absence of melanin in the epidermis (Mollet I. et al., 2007)

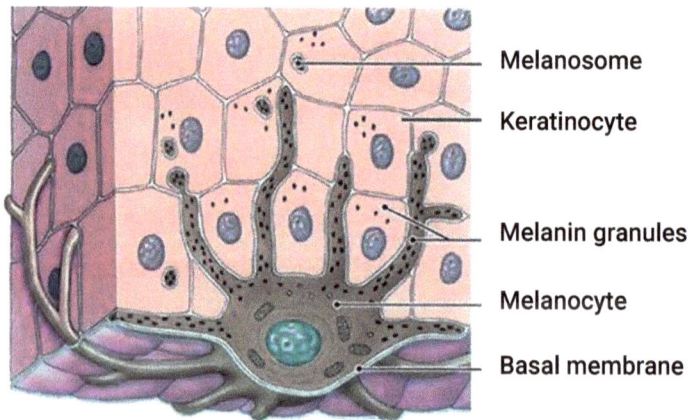

Melanosome

Keratinocyte

Melanin granules

Melanocyte

Basal membrane

Figure II-4-1. Distribution of melanosomes in the epidermis

Skincare practitioners are most frequently faced with excessive melanin accumulation, i.e., hyperpigmentation — both primary, arising on unaltered skin (freckles, melasma, pigmentation due to hormonal and metabolic disorders, etc.), and secondary, developing after inflammatory processes (acne, trauma, surgery, aesthetic interventions).

4.1. Diagnosis

The amount, depth, and density of melanin distribution characterize pigmented lesions. Depending on the pigment depth, all lesions are divided into:

1. **Epidermal:**
   - Freckles
   - Lentigo
   - Seborrheic keratosis
   - Spotted nevus
   - Café-au-lait stains
   - Epidermal melasma
2. **Dermal:**
   - Nevus of Ota (cutaneous ocular melanosis)
   - Nevus of Ito (similar to Nevus of Ota, but localizes in the neck and upper torso)
   - Mongolian spot (common for mongoloid and negroid individuals; in light-skinned individuals, it occurs in only 1–10% of cases)
   - Dermal melasma
3. **Dermo-epidermal (mixed):**
   - Congenital melanocytic nevus
   - Acquired melanocytic nevus
   - Post-inflammatory hyperpigmentation
   - Becker's nevus
   - Mixed melasma

Sometimes, pigmentary lesions are easy to diagnose by simple inspection: epidermal — brown, dermal — blue or gray, and mixed — heterogeneous brown–gray color with dark and light areas within a single spot.

In addition, pigmentary lesions differ according to the distribution of pigment (intracellular *vs.* extracellular), can be congenital or acquired, limited or widespread, and according to the nature of the pigment — it can be not only melanin, but also silver (argyria) and iron oxide (hemosiderosis).

Melasma is a particular challenge, as it is an acquired hypomelanosis located on the face that occurs most often in women with skin phototype III–V. Melanin in melasma can be found at the epidermis as well as dermis (Lai D. et al., 2022).

4.2. How dye lasers and IPL work

Melanin is the primary target for pigmentary defects. Ideally, dye lasers should generate radiation absorbed only by melanin, with minimal absorption by hemoglobin or water. However, melanin's absorption spectrum overlaps with these chromophores' absorption spectra. The 630–1100 nm wavelength range is considered relatively selective for melanin exposure (Araghi F. et al., 2022), where radiation penetrates well into the skin and is preferentially absorbed by melanin relative to oxyhemoglobin (**Fig. II-4-2**).

Light energy absorption by melanin decreases as the radiation wavelength increases, but longer wavelengths allow deeper penetration into the skin. At the same time, shorter wavelengths can damage pigment cells with relatively low energy, and longer wavelengths, while penetrating deeper, need more energy to cause damage to melanosomes. Thus, it is impossible to achieve an isolated effect on melanin through wavelength selection alone (optical selectivity).

Therefore, another challenge arises — delivering the greatest number of photons to the target chromophore before they are absorbed by competing chromophores close to the target. This is possible via optimal selection of the pulse duration and the radiation energy parameters.

Since melanin and melanin-filled melanosomes are very small, less prolonged heating is required to destroy them than, for example, to coagulate blood vessels. As we have already mentioned, to achieve selective laser action, the pulse duration should be at least equal to, and

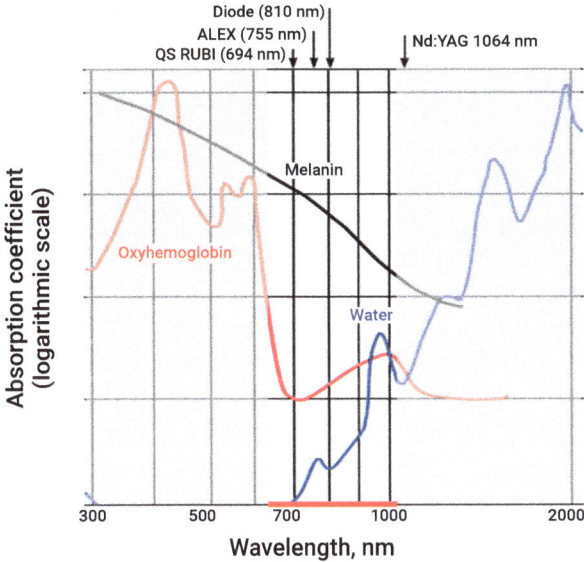

Figure II-4-2. The 630–1100 nm wavelength range is considered relatively selective for melanin exposure, because radiation penetrates well into the skin and is preferentially absorbed by melanin

ideally several times shorter than, the target structure's TRT. Otherwise, it does not have time to cool down, and significant heating spreads to the adjacent non-target tissues, causing their thermal damage.

The TRT of melanosomes ranges from 50 to 250 ns; thus, for their effective and safe destruction, the pulse duration of laser exposure should be in the nanosecond or even picosecond range. At the same time, the pulse energy should be high enough to destroy the target without overheating the surrounding structures.

4.3. Appliances for the treatment of pigmentary disorders

In light of the considerations given above, today, pigmentary lesions are primarily treated with Q-switched (QS) lasers that generate ns and ps pulses. Destruction of melanin with ultrashort-pulsed lasers occurs not only due to photothermolysis but also owing to the photoacoustic

Table II-4-1. Types of laser devices for the treatment of pigmented skin pathology

SELECTIVE SHORT-PULSED LASERS (NANO- AND PICO-SECOND LASERS)	SELECTIVE LONG-PULSED LASERS AND IPL DEVICES	FRACTIONAL LASERS	LASER DERMABRASION
• Copper vapor laser (511 nm) • QS KTP (532 nm) • QS RUBY (694 nm) • QS ALEX (755/785 nm) • QS Nd:YAG (1064 nm) • Fractional tips for picosecond lasers (532, 755, 1064 nm)	• KTP (532 nm) • PDL 585, 595 nm) • ALEX (755 nm) • IPL (560–1200 nm)	**Non-ablative fractional lasers:** • 1540–1550 nm **Ablative fractional lasers:** • Er:YSGG (2770 nm) • Er:YAG (2940 nm) • CO_2 (10,600 nm)	• Er:YSGG (2770 nm) • Er:YAG (2940 nm) • CO_2 (10,600 nm)

effect: rapid heating of tissues leads to the emergence of shockwaves that "break" pigment granules into individual fragments, which are then utilized by macrophages. The shorter the pulse duration, the more pronounced the photomechanical effect, and the lesser the photothermal effect (Gaffey M.M., Johnson A.B., 2024).

Fractional ablative and non-ablative lasers are also used to remove pigmented lesions (including a separate line of work to enhance penetration of depigmenting agents from the area of work), as well as IPL sources with filters to target the pigmented pathology (**Table II-4-1**).

The choice of laser will be determined primarily by the pigment depth.

■ **Superficial epidermal lesions** can be removed using laser radiation that is highly absorbed by melanin, as the risk of competitive interaction is low. These can be both long-pulsed and short-pulsed lasers, as well as IPL systems:
  – Long-pulsed lasers: 511, 532, 585/595, 694, 755 nm
  – QS lasers: 532, 755, 785, 1064 nm
  – IPL: 560–1200 nm

- **Superficial epidermal pigment lesions with keratosis (seborrheic or actinic keratosis)** require the destruction of both pigment and hyperkeratotic lesion; thus, the leading method will be ablative photothermolysis by fractional Er:YAG and CO_2 lasers.
- **Dermal pigmentation** requires high-energy short pulses (of nano- and picosecond duration) generated by QS lasers at 755 and 1064 nm. Resurfacing is contraindicated in the case of dermal defects.

Green light
Effects and targets
Green light's penetrating power is relatively low, and its effect is limited only to the epidermis. Therefore, lasers emitting in the green part of the spectrum can be used to treat superficial epidermal hyperpigmentation (epidermal melasma, lentigo, freckles, café-au-lait spots, and Becker's nevi).

Devices
- **Copper vapor laser (511 nm).** Short nanosecond pulses make it possible to produce both photoacoustic and photothermal destruction. The first mechanism mainly results in the destruction of melanin, and the second destroys melanocytes. By varying the power and duration of exposure of the pigment defect, it is possible to regulate the ratio between these mechanisms. However, as 511-nm radiation cannot penetrate deep layers, it can only be used to remove superficial defects.
- **Long-pulsed KTP, QS KTP (532 nm).** Radiation at this wavelength is well absorbed by both melanin and hemoglobin and acts on the superficial skin layers. After exposure to QS KTP, destruction of melanosomes and more pronounced damage to melanocytes in general is noted, in place of which the formation of new cells producing normal amounts of pigment is registered. The use of low energy density is recommended. However, some studies have shown that long-pulsed QS KTP lasers are more effective in eliminating superficial pigmentation than short-pulsed QS devices.

Impact features

These lasers are undesirable in people with dark skin phototypes, because the radiation within the green part of the spectrum is extremely actively absorbed by melanin, potentially causing burns and additional changes in pigmentation (both hypo- and hyperpigmentation). Even in case of an initial successful result with their use, subsequent recurrence of pigmentation defects is possible.

Since waves within this spectral range are also well absorbed by hemoglobin, purpura and small bruises may appear after using these lasers. Usually, they disappear 1–2 weeks after the procedure, but in some cases post-inflammatory hyperpigmentation may develop in place of hemangiomas. Therefore, before treating large areas of skin, experts recommend performing test procedures on small areas.

Yellow light
Effects and targets

The penetrating power of yellow light is higher than that of green light but is still low. Therefore, these lasers are also mainly used for epidermal defects.

Devices: long-pulsed PDL (585, 595 nm).

Impact features

As radiation at 585 and 595 nm wavelengths is well absorbed mainly by hemoglobin, PDLs are the "gold standard" for treating vascular lesions. Still, it is also absorbed by melanin and is sometimes used for superficial pigment lesions. However, PDL is particularly beneficial in melasma because increased vascularization plays an important role in its pathogenesis (Dai X. et al., 2022). Receptors for the vascular growth factors VEGF-1 and VEGF-2 have been found on the surface of melanocytes, which can influence cell activity; hence, acting on the vascular component can reduce stimulation of melanocyte activity and lessen pigmentation.

Red light
Effects and targets
The red wavelengths penetrate deeper than the green wavelengths, allowing them to be used to correct both epidermal and dermal pigmentations.

Devices: QS RUBY (694 nm), QS ALEX (755 nm).

QS RUBY (694 nm). RUBY laser is used to correct a wide range of hyperpigmentations (melasma, melanocytic nevi, lentigo, café-au-lait spots, nevi of Ota, chloasma, Becker's nevi, etc.). At the same time, the procedures carry a relatively low risk of adverse side effects (most of which were noted when using the RUBY laser for treating the nevi of Ota). It can be assumed that the latter is due to the higher energy levels used for therapy in dermal hyperpigmentation cases. This hypothesis is confirmed by the fact that, even when the gentler fractional QS RUBY is used to treat superficial pigmentation in people with light skin phototypes, high energy densities significantly increase the incidence of adverse events. Specialists thus suggest careful patient selection and more gentle procedures.

QS ALEX (755 nm). Melanin absorbs ALEX-emitted radiation less intensively than that produced by RUBY laser, so it can be used in patients with darker skin. However, experts recommend using a relatively low dose and limiting the number of treatments. Nano- and picosecond QS ALEX lasers can be used to remove lentigos, benign melanocytic lesions, café-au-lait spots, nevi of Oto, and melasma.

Impact features
Unlike green light-generating devices, these lasers do not produce bruising, as red-band radiation is much less absorbed by hemoglobin. However, while the damage to melanocytes will be substantial, recurrences are also possible.

Near-IR light
Effects and targets
The absorption intensity of near-IR radiation by melanin is relatively low (less than for the green and red bands). Still, other chromophores, such as hemoglobin and water, absorb it even less intensively.

This accounts for the high penetrating ability of this radiation and the possibility of its use for treating deep dermal pigmentary defects.

Devices: QS Nd:YAG (1064 nm).

Impact features

Ultrashort-pulsed (nano- and picosecond) 1064-nm radiation causes fragmentation and disintegration of melanin granules, sublethal damage to melanosomes, and release of pigment into the cytoplasm of cells. The low absorbance of radiation by melanin allows the use of low-dose radiation produced by QS Nd:YAG laser in people with dark skin phototypes — it is poorly absorbed by the epidermal pigment, which reduces the risk of hypopigmentation and burns. Therefore, although in general 1064-nm radiation is less impactful on pigmentary defects, QS Nd:YAG laser is the primary choice in people with III–V phototypes.

Another feature of QS Nd:YAG laser is its complex action: although melanin most actively absorbs its radiation, it also acts on hemoglobin and water molecules. Therefore, along with pigment destruction, vessel coagulation can be observed (which, for example, is relevant in the case of excessive vascularization related to melasma). Damage to collagen is also achieved, resulting in dermal remodeling, rejuvenation, and even skin tone. A combination of these effects is used in the so-called "laser tinting" procedure, which is popular in Asian countries.

In general, relatively long intervals between sessions and their limited number are recommended for treating pigmented lesions. Thus, the following exposure parameters are most frequently used for melasma correction: energy density — 2–4 J/cm^2, pulse duration — 5–12 ms, spot size — 6 mm, 5–10 sessions at 7-day intervals.

IPL
Effects and targets

Energy in the wavelength range generated by IPL devices (500–1200 nm) is absorbed by all major skin chromophores: melanin, hemoglobin, and water. Special light filters are used for more targeted exposure. For example, 500–550-nm filters can be used for epidermal pigment lesions, and long-wave filters are recommended for deeper melanin depots.

Impact features

The energy of intense pulsed light is distributed among different chromophores, reducing its impact on individual targets. It is therefore necessary to increase the intensity to achieve a pronounced effect on specific structures. Still, this strategy is fraught with undesirable side effects: high energy densities are associated with the risk of burns and post-inflammatory hyperpigmentation in patients with dark skin phototypes. Therefore, the indications for IPL application are primarily superficial epidermal pigmentary disorders, although such procedures are often less effective than when using lasers emitting light in the green and red parts of the spectrum.

Laser resurfacing and fractional photothermolysis
Effects and targets

The main target for laser resurfacing and fractional photothermolysis is water, and since it is present in all skin cells and structures, not only melanocytes but all tissues are damaged. As a result, laser resurfacing is rarely used to remove pigmentary lesions and is applied only in hyperkeratotic formations. However, even in this case, fractional lasers are preferred. The depth of their effect is adjustable: fractional lasers can be used for superficial and deep pigmentary disorders, in particular for lentigo, melasma, Becker's nevus, nevus of Ota, seborrheic keratosis, and post-inflammatory hyperpigmentation.

Devices and exposure features

For ablative fractional photothermolysis (with damage to the *stratum corneum*):

- CO_2 (10,600 nm)
- Er:YAG (2940 nm)

In ablative fractional photothermolysis, due to the high absorbance of 2940 nm and 10,600 nm radiation by water, it almost immediately evaporates even from those cells containing very little moisture (the *stratum corneum*). Although fractional procedures are less traumatic than laser resurfacing, they are also associated with a risk of post-inflammatory hyperpigmentation. Some experts recommend using this method only to remove small pigment lesions such as lentigo, seborrheic keratosis, or hyperpigmentation resistant to other types of therapy.

For non-ablative fractional photothermolysis (the *stratum corneum* remains intact):
- **Diode laser (1440 nm)** for complex melasma therapy:
  - three treatments of low-intensity exposure with 3-week intervals
  - whitening creams (in the morning, based on ascorbic and kojic acid; in the evening, based on 0.025% tretinoin)
  - weekly peels with 20% salicylic acid
- **Fractionated Nd:YAG laser (1440 nm)** for nevus of Ota resistant to Nd:YAG (1064 nm)
- **Erbium laser (1550 nm):** The following exposure parameters are used for melasma: MTZ density — 2000–2500 per cm^2, 6–10 mJ per microbeam; 3–4 sessions with an interval of 1–2 months. Good results (35–50% improvement on average) are achieved, and undesirable side effects are rare.
- **Thulium laser (1927 nm):** This radiation is more readily absorbed by water than the radiation emitted by other non-ablative lasers, so it is more effective in damaging epidermal pigments.

Non-ablative fractional photothermolysis is performed using radiation in the 1300–2000 nm wavelength range. This spectrum has a lower absorption coefficient than the radiation of ablative lasers and provides heating of epidermis and dermis structures up to 45–90 °C (coagulation). It is recommended for the correction of dermal and mixed pigment formations, uneven skin tone, and melasma.

Since melasma formation (and, according to some reports, post-inflammatory hyperpigmentation) also has vascular causes, some specialists recommend combining non-ablative fractional photothermolysis with selective photothermolysis by PDL (510 nm) or KTP (532 nm) for better results.

4.4. Effectiveness of laser therapy

Clinical experience shows that different pigmentary disorders respond diffretently to laser treatment (**Table II-4-2** and **Table II-4-3**).

Table II-4-2. Expected response to laser treatment

GOOD RESPONSE	MODERATE RESPONSE	VARIABLE RESPONSE	CONFLICTING RESULTS
Lentigo, freckles, seborrheic keratosis, nevus of Ota, nevus of Ito	Melasma and post-inflamma-tory hyperpig-mentation	Café-au-lait spots, spotted nevus, Becker's nevus	Congenital and acquired melanocytic nevi (risk of incomplete destruction and removal of deep-seated nevus cells)

Table II-4-3. Estimated efficacy depending on the localization of pigment lesions

DEVICE	LOCALIZATION		
	EPIDERMIS	EPIDERMIS AND DERMIS	DERMIS
QS copper vapor lasers (511 nm)	+++	++	+
Long-pulsed KTP, QS KTP (532 nm)	+++	++	+
QS RUBY (694 nm)	+++	+++	++
QS ALEX (755 nm)	++	+++	++
QS Nd:YAG (1064 nm)	+	+++	+++
IPL	+++	+++	+
Ablative fractional photothermolysis	+++	+	+
Non-ablative fractional photothermolysis	+	++	+++

A separate issue with using lasers to remove melanocytic nevi is the need to be sure that these tumors are indeed benign. There is currently no evidence to suggest that laser exposure can induce malignant cell degeneration, but there is a considerable body of data related to the removal of pre-existing undiagnosed skin cancer using inadequate protocols, followed by more growth or problems stemming from late diagnosis.

Therefore, prior to the removal of pigmented lesions, both clinical examination and dermatoscopy are required. In any suspicious cases, histologic examination should be performed, and preferably other methods of pigmentary defect removal should be utilized.

If the decision to proceed with the laser removal is made, the formation should be excised with a scalpel or scissors, the tissue should be sent for histologic examination, and only when the results are obtained the remaining pigment should be removed by laser. Still, even in this case, problems may arise, as the excised tissue may not include a malignant focus, leading to erroneous diagnosis. Therefore, where there are doubts, it is better not to attempt laser removal of pigmentary formations.

4.5. Laser therapy for hypopigmentation disorders

Hypomelanoses include vitiligo, post-inflammatory hypopigmentation, idiopathic hypomelanosis, pigmentless nevus, etc., whereby those resulting from the reduction or disappearance of pigment are more resistant to therapy. Their appearance may be associated with a decrease in the number of melanocytes and their normal content in the presence of a defect in the melanogenesis system or melanosome transport.

There are several options for the laser treatment of vitiligo (Post N.F. et al., 2022). In the case of generalized vitiligo, patients are offered depigmentation of areas where normal skin color is preserved, using topical bleaching agents or lasers to eliminate excess pigmentation (e.g., QS RUBY, QS ALEX). However, restoring skin pigmentation in the affected areas is more common. For this purpose, laser resurfacing or ablative fractional photothermolysis with Er:YAG or CO_2 lasers and microdermabrasion are used. Their aim is to eliminate defective areas and stimulate the formation of new normally functioning melanocytes.

Another mode of hypopigmentation therapy involves stimulating melanocyte migration and proliferation. For this purpose, devices emitting in the UV range are used, particularly excimer lasers (308 nm). The effectiveness of helium–neon lasers (632.8 nm) in this context is also being studied. Despite being in the red spectrum, the radiation emitted by these lasers also has a stimulating effect on melanocytes.

Light-based technologies do not always provide 100% and safe removal of pigment spots, but they are effective for almost all types of dyschromia. Understanding the capabilities of modern device-based methods will aid in a more correct laser selection depending on the type of disorder and will increase the procedure effectiveness and safety.

More information on the treatment of pigmentation disorders can be found in the *Pigmentation in Cosmetic Dermatology & Skincare Practice* book.

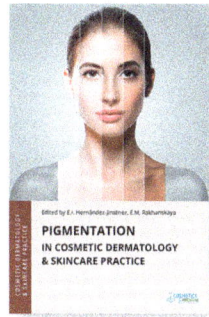

Edited by E.I. Hernández-Jiménez, E.M. Rákhmetova

PIGMENTATION
IN COSMETIC DERMATOLOGY
& SKINCARE PRACTICE

Chapter 5
Scars

A scar is newly formed connective tissue accompanied by destruction of the dermis. According to their etiology, scars are categorized as post-traumatic, postoperative, or post-inflammatory (including post-acne). Striae can also be considered scars.

There are many methods of scar revision. However, it is essential to realize that it is currently impossible to completely remove scar deformities. Aesthetic treatment only reduces the severity of clinical symptoms, which lessens discomfort and makes the scar less noticeable. There is no single standard protocol for scar correction due to the wide clinical diversity of scar types and presentations (Chen S.X. et al., 2022).

5.1. Diagnosis

When choosing a treatment strategy, it is necessary to consider the scar's type and maturity, which have prognostic value for the treatment outcome and affect the likelihood of recurrence (Xiao A., Ettefagh L., 2022). For this reason, at the initial consultation, the physician should fully assess the clinical picture, determining the degree of severity of all scar features in each case (**Table II-5-1**). The clinical picture should be monitored during treatment, and its dynamics should be tracked.

The totality of all clinical features, considering their degree of expression, allows us to determine the type of scar and its maturity stage. This was the basis for the clinical and morphologic classification, which, from a practical point of view, is the most convenient for use in clinical practice (**Table II-5-2**).

Clinical and morphologic classifications make it possible to determine the best course of treatment with reasonable confidence (the benefits of different methods or their combinations, and the order of their application) and predict the scar revision results.

Table II-5-1. Clinical signs of scars, degrees of their severity

SIGN	DEGREE OF SEVERITY
Subjective sensations in the scar area	• Absent • Paresthesias • Itching (intermittent or persistent) • Pain
Vascular component	• Absent — pale scar color • Minor — pale pink scar color • Moderate — pink scar color • Expressed — scar color from bright red to bluish–buggy
Scar tissue density	• Reduced — flabbiness • Normal — close to normal skin density • Elevated — exceeding that of normal skin density • Significantly tense — cartilage-like tissue
Tissue relief in relation to the surrounding skin	• Depression • On the same level • Elevation — moderate (up to 0.5 cm) or significant (more than 0.5 cm)
Pigmentation in the scar area	• De- and hypopigmentation • Normal • Hyperpigmentation

Table II-5-2. Clinical and morphologic classification of scars

MATURITY	CHARACTERISTIC CLINICAL SIGNS	SCAR TYPE
Mature scars	• The clinical picture is stable, or changes are minor (minimal, very slow, externally barely noticeable) • No tendency for scar tissue volume increase • Vascular component is absent or weakly expressed (pale or pale pink coloration) • Tissue density is decreased, normal, or moderately increased • No superficial tissue tension • Subjective sensations in the scar area are absent	• Normotrophic scars • Hypo- and atrophic scars • Hypertrophic scars in • Scars in the regression stage (at least two years old)

Continued on p. 104

MATURITY	CHARACTERISTIC CLINICAL SIGNS	SCAR TYPE
Immature scars	• Visible dynamics of the clinical picture over time • Tendency for the scar tissue volume to increase • High sensitivity to external influences • Subjective sensations in the scar area with varying degrees of severity • Vascular component (red to livid-blue coloration) • Tissue density from normal to significantly elevated • Surface tissue tension with a pearlescent sheen is possible	• Fresh scars, up to 12 months old • Hypertrophic scars up to two years old and small keloids* • Large and multiple keloids

* Hypertrophic scars (1–2 years old) and small keloids are considered together, as their clinical manifestations are similar. These types of scars can be reliably distinguished using histologic examination or ultrasound, which is rarely used in the routine clinical practice.

5.2. How lasers work when used for scar revision

Laser scar revision includes several approaches based on applying different types of laser radiation. Each radiation type affects a specific chromophore in tissues, producing different photobiological effects. The indications and results of using different lasers in scar correction will differ.

There are several advantages of laser scar revision over other methods:

- ■ It is possible to carry out complex treatment by combining several types of laser devices and applying them sequentially on the same scar, potentiating the effect of revision.
- ■ It is possible to treat scars of any localization, including areas of the body with active movements (for example, in the projection of joints), which does not require the patient to limit mobility.
- ■ No pronounced systemic effects on the body.
- ■ Possibility of use in children.

It should be considered that the laser therapy reduces clinical manifestations but not the scar area, which can be achieved only by surgery.

Laser therapy for scars includes:

- Vascular coagulation
- Laser dermabrasion
- Fractional photothermolysis
- Hyperpigmentation removal

5.3. Laser therapy for scars

5.3.1. Laser coagulation of vessels

- KTP (532 nm)
- PDL (575, 595 nm)

Oxyhemoglobin is the target chromophore. The mechanism of action is related to the photothermal effect on vascular coagulation.

The objective is removing **the vascular component in the scar** and its pallor. Reducing vascularization contributes to eliminating hyperemia of hypo- and atrophic scars, and improving their appearance. In the case of immature scars, vessel coagulation accelerates scar tissue maturation, which clinically manifests not only in the elimination of the vascular component and pale tissue but also in the disappearance of subjective sensations, as well as scar density and excessive volume reduction.

The mechanism of immature scar improvement has yet to be established. Several theories exist, one of which suggests local tissue ischemization due to decreased nutrition, which reduces cell functional activity and the amount of immature collagen matrix.

Indications for using the laser vascular coagulation are:

1. **Immature scarring:**
   - Fresh scars with a pronounced vascular component, a tendency to hypertrophic growth, and presence of subjective sensations
   - Hypertrophic scars that are up to two years old and small keloids
   - Large and multiple keloids (as a part of complex scar therapy)
2. **Mature scars** with vascular congestion

5.3.2. Laser resurfacing

- Er:YAG (2940 nm)
- CO_2 (10,600 nm)

The target chromophore for mid- and far-IR radiation is water. Exposure to this laser radiation causes photothermal effect in the form of ablation (i.e., vaporization of the surface tissue layers) due to its high absorption by water. At the same time, a wound surface is formed, i.e., this method is traumatic. The ablation depth depends on the type of laser used, energy parameters, and the number of passes over the same area. These factors are selected individually and can vary across different treatment areas to target the formation of surface relief.

The result is a smoothing of the uneven topography between the scar tissue and the surrounding skin.

For a long time, only hypo- and atrophic mature scars, as well as hypertrophic scars in the regression stage (more than two years old), were considered as indications for laser dermabrasion because it seemed that exposure of immature scars was associated with a high risk of pathologic scarring recurrence. However, since the approaches to fractional exposure are being revised, so are the approaches to laser resurfacing.

5.3.3. Fractional photothermolysis

The main expected effect of fractional photothermolysis is the reorganization of scar tissue. This involves inhibiting the formation of malformed collagen, destroying excess collagen, and stimulating new collagen formation. Due to the reorganization of scar tissue, there is an indirect improvement of color and smoothing of borders with normal skin.

The indications for fractional photothermolysis can include all types of scars, i.e., they are quite diverse, and so are the effects obtained. Recent studies suggest that there is no need to wait for scar maturation, and fractional ablative treatment of immature scar tissue can (and should) be performed to reduce the risk of pathologic scar formation. It is believed that laser microdamage modulates the wound healing process and "pushes" the treated scar tissue to mature along a more normotrophic pathway. Moreover, some studies have shown the effectiveness of preoperative skin treatment targeting the area where surgery will be performed to normalize and improve the healing process after surgery.

5.3.4. Laser removal of hyperpigmentation in the scar area

Laser pigment removal is used in case of hyperpigmentation, as hypopigmentation and depigmentation are not amenable to laser therapy and can be corrected by camouflage tattooing only.

To destroy pigment and eliminate the hyperpigmentation that is sometimes seen in hypo-, atrophic, and normotrophic scars, the following lasers are used:

- QS Nd:YAG (1064 nm)
- QS RUBY (694 nm)
- QS ALEX (755 nm)

The target chromophore is melanin. The result is mediated by a photomechanical effect that destroys excess pigment, eliminates hyperpigmentation in the scar projection, and aligns its color with the surrounding skin.

Indications: mature scars with hyperpigmentation.

The possibilities of using different lasers depending on the type of scar are provided in **Table II-5-3** and **Table II-5-4**.

Table II-5-3. Laser therapy for mature scar revision

SCAR TYPE	CLINICAL MANIFESTATION	THERAPY	EXPECTED EFFECT
Hypo- and atrophic scars	• Relief: depression, lack of volume • Tissue turgor: decreased • Congestive hyperemia • Color: hypo- and depigmentation **(should not be treated!)**	Fractional photother-molysis	Tissue turgor increase and relief optimization
		Laser derma-brasion	Relief leveling
		Laser vascular coagulation	Elimination of congestive hyperemia and color optimization

Continued on p. 108

SCAR TYPE	CLINICAL MANIFESTATION	THERAPY	EXPECTED EFFECT
Normotrophic scars	• Altered tissue structure and surface: folding, smoothness • Dyschromia: hypo-, de-, and hyperpigmentation	Fractional photothermolysis	Optimization of tissue structure, smoothing the "scar–healthy skin" boundaries
		Laser removal of hyperpigmentation	Removal of excess pigment
Hypertrophic scars in regression (more than two years old)	• Relief: elevation, excess volume • Tissue turgor: elevated • Slight hyperemia (residual vascular component)	Fractional photothermolysis	Decreased tissue density and reduced scar volume
		Laser dermabrasion	Removal of excess scar tissue — smoothing the relief
		Laser vascular coagulation	Elimination of hyperemia and color optimization

Table II-5-4. Possibilities of using laser methods in the immature scars revision

SCAR TYPE	CLINICAL SIGNS	REVISION-METHOD	EXPECTED EFFECT
Fresh scars (up to 12 months old)	• Subjective feelings • Hyperemia • Relief: there may be irregularity or growth of scar tissue	Laser vascular coagulation	Elimination of subjective sensations and hyperemia
		Fractional photothermolysis, laser resurfacing	Suppression of excessive collagen formation, smoothing the "scar–healthy skin" boundaries
Hypertrophic scars (1–2 years old), small keloids	• Relief: elevation, excess volume • Hyperemia • Tissue turgor: significantly elevated • Subjective feelings	Laser vascular coagulation	Elimination of subjective sensations, reduction of erythema, reduction of tissue density, reduction of scar volume, prevention of recurrence
		Fractional photothermolysis, laser resurfacing	Destruction of excess collagen — reducing tissue density and volume

5.4. Laser scar therapy

Table II-5-5 presents the stages of the conventional scar laser revision.

Table II-5-5. Stages of the scar laser revision

STEP	DESCRIPTION
1	Evaluation of the clinical picture and the degree of symptom severity, to determine the type of scar.
2	Identification of the leading symptom in the overall clinical picture. In **immature scars**, the presence of subjective sensations at any degree of severity is always considered as a leading symptom (it is a marker of the risk of pathologic scarring and recurrence).* In patients with **normotrophic scars**, when low degree of expression is noted for all clinical symptoms, the decision primarily pertains to the expediency of corrective therapy.*
3	Selection of the laser treatment for the correction of the leading symptom; evaluation of the influence of the selected type of radiation on the other clinical symptoms.
4	Performing procedures until the expected effect is obtained. In **immature scars**, attainment of negative dynamics (increasing subjective sensations) or their absence is an indication for the need to include medical therapeutic methods (local administration of glucocorticosteroids, lysosomal enzymes).*
5	Reassessment of the clinical picture from the perspective of the dynamics, the degree of symptom severity, and the leading symptom. In case of **immature scars**, regular dynamic examinations (at 2-week intervals at least*) are mandatory.
6	If necessary, another laser method aimed at the correction of the next highlighted leading symptom is employed. In case of **immature scars**, switching to another laser method is possible only after the subjective sensations* have been completely eliminated.
	Repeat steps 4–6 until the optimal aesthetic result is obtained.

* Key differences between treatment protocols. Immature scar therapy always requires great caution and responsibility from the doctor because the development of such scars is unpredictable. It is mandatory to monitor the dynamics at least once every two weeks and, if necessary, to change the treatment strategy.

5.5. When to start scar therapy

Previously, it was believed that if the scar was in an unstable state, it was impossible to tell whether scarring would be physiological or pathological, so early intervention was deemed risky and unjustified.

However, today, many experts advocate for early intervention as it allows the "direction" of the maturation process to proceed along the normotrophic pathway.

5.6. Comprehensive approach to scar management

Despite the wide possibilities and high efficiency of laser methods of scar revision as monotherapy and when the lasers are combined, there are several clinical situations in which it is necessary to add other methods, bearing mind the following guidelines:

■ Intracutaneous injections of corticosteroids (diprospan, kenalog) should precede laser therapy in pronounced subjective sensations or progressive scar growth with a significant volume of scar tissue.

■ Topical medications (silicone patch, fermencol gel, etc.) can be used between laser sessions if the scar is in a permanently traumatized area and therefore poorly amenable.

Treatment of large and numerous keloids requires a comprehensive approach. Still, it should be noted that surgeons in specialized hospitals typically treat such scars. If skincare practitioners choose to treat this category of patients, they must recognize that such pathology is associated with impaired immunological and endocrine status. As a result, it is necessary to refer patients for consultations with related specialists and, if abnormalities are detected, to jointly conduct therapy (Leszczynski R. et al., 2022).

The management of large and numerous keloid scars should be performed gradually in small areas (up to about 10 cm^2). Only after obtaining a positive result in one area should the correction in other areas be carried out.

In some cases, surgical revision is preferred, whereby laser methods are omitted or are employed after surgical intervention. This advice applies to cases characterized by:

- Possibility of excising the scar and creating a smaller defect
- Scar plasty with a skin flap associated with a low risk of pathologic scarring
- Possibility of moving the scar from a visible to a hidden area
- Elimination of scar adhesions with the underlying tissues, causing its retraction into the skin
- Foreign body in the scar tissue

It should be remembered that laser therapy includes several steps, the results are evaluated only after several months, and the effect build-up lasts up to a year. The more pronounced the scar deformity, the greater the opportunities for revision, and the more significant the visual result will be. The less pronounced the clinical symptoms are at the beginning, the less visible the changes are after correction. Naturally, this can cause patient dissatisfaction, so it is important to discuss the therapy options and likely outcomes in detail at the initial consultation.

More information on the scar treatment is provided in the *Scars and Striae in Cosmetic Dermatology & Skincare Practice* book.

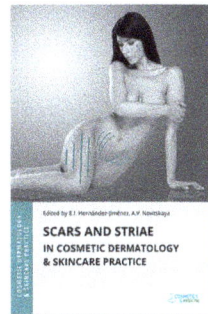

Edited by E.I. Hernández-Jiménez, A.V. Novitskaya

SCARS AND STRIAE
IN COSMETIC DERMATOLOGY
& SKINCARE PRACTICE

Chapter 6
Acne and psoriasis

Acne (acne vulgaris) is one of the most common inflammatory skin diseases, affecting up to 85% of adolescents and young adults. In about 65%, 43%, and 15% of these cases, rashes persist into the third, fourth, and fifth decade of life. Age-related acne occurs predominantly in women.

Conventional treatments for this condition include topical and systemic retinoids and antibiotics, azelaic acid, benzoyl peroxide, traditional external agents (salicylic acid, levomycetin, resorcinol), and other topical preparations. In addition, women are prescribed combined oral contraceptives and androgen receptor inhibitors. Unfortunately, however, these methods do not always result in improvement. As they are also associated with undesirable side effects, the search for alternative approaches to acne treatment is ongoing. In this context, phototherapy — not only with low-intensity light but also with high-intensity light — has emerged as a promising candidate.

Acne treatment using lasers and IPL is gradually gaining popularity in skincare practice. Even though these approaches, as well as other light-based methods, have been in use for more than twenty years, there still needs to be a consensus among experts on this issue. However, due to the growing body of research into the possibility of using these approaches as a monotherapy, it is possible to better assess their effectiveness. Some researchers argue that, at present, light-based methods are still insufficiently effective because they facilitate inflammation resolution at a certain stage of the process, but do not guarantee acne-free skin for a long period of time. Others believe that these methods are quite effective and, in combination with topical therapy, can become the basis for acne treatment (Barbaric J. et al., 2016).

6.1. How lasers and IPL work for acne

Light-based methods work by affecting certain targets in tissues that absorb radiation. In acne, such a target should be the sebaceous gland. However, the sebaceous gland does not contain substances that could serve as specific chromophores for implementing the principle of selective photothermolysis. Therefore, the therapeutic result is achieved indirectly.

Targets for phototherapy can be:

- Melanosomes, which are located at the mouth of the sebaceous hair follicle
- Melanosomes of the hair shaft
- Nearby blood vessels
- Endogenous porphyrins — substances that are produced by *Cutibacterium acnes*
- Sebum in the sebaceous gland

Depending on the type of radiation used and the parameters of its delivery, light-based technologies mainly produce a photobiological effect or a combination of effects in tissues.

- **Photochemical effect:** It is realized due to the effect of radiation on endogenous or exogenous (their formation is stimulated by photosensitizer) porphyrins, which are produced directly by *Cutibacterium acnes* bacteria. Under the influence of radiation, porphyrins decompose with the release of ROS, and this has a destructive effect on the bacteria themselves, i.e., the bactericidal impact of the photochemical effect is manifested.
- **Photothermal effect:** When tissues around the sebaceous gland are heated, local immune response is stimulated, resulting in an immunomodulatory effect. Thermal damage reduces the volume of the sebaceous gland and its contents due to the effect on water and sebum.
- Although the significance of vascular coagulation in acne is not fully understood, based on theoretical assumptions, the sebaceous gland's nutrition worsens due to vascular coagulation, reducing its functional activity. This, in turn, leads to a decrease in the inflammatory response of tissues. Hair removal

also contributes to the inflammatory process reduction, most likely due to the improvement in sebum evacuation.

- **Photomechanical effect:** Shockwave destroys the bonds between keratinocytes, due to which the hyperkeratotic wall around the orifice is removed, the evacuation of sebum from the duct is facilitated, and anaerobic conditions are eliminated, yielding a bacteriostatic effect.

The intensity of photobiological effects is determined by radiation parameters: wavelength (or range of wavelengths), intensity (energy flux), and pulse duration.

6.2. Phototherapy devices

Classic phototherapy with blue and/or red light

Low-intensity blue and red light is used to treat mild to moderate acne (Ablon G., 2018).

Radiation of 407–420 nm wavelength (in the violet–blue part of the spectrum) is absorbed by porphyrins (protoporphyrin IX and coproporphyrin), which are produced by *C. acnes* (**Fig. II-6-1**). In this case, their excitation and subsequent formation of singlet oxygen and active radicals that damage cells (phototoxic effect) occur (Diogo M.L.G. et al., 2021; Sadowska M. et al., 2021). Red light is absorbed by porphyrins much less intensely, but it penetrates deeper, has an anti-inflammatory effect (induces the release of cytokines from macrophages), and accelerates healing. Therefore, red light is usually not used separately for acne treatment, only to reduce the severity of inflammation, but in combination with blue light, it yields a very good effect.

No significant contraindications or serious side effects have been identified in this type of therapy. LED devices are mainly used to produce blue and red light.

KTP

KTP emits light with a wavelength of 532 nm, which belongs to the green part of the spectrum. It penetrates deeper than blue light, although not as deeply as red, but is better absorbed by *C. acnes*

BLUE LIGHT

Epidermis

Flavins | Porphyrins | Nitrosated proteins | Opsin = G protein | Cytochrome c oxidase

TRPV1

Dermis

ROS | NO | CAMK II | Modulation of mitochondrial activity

Nucleus

Cell survival, growth, regulation of inflammation | Cells differentiation, anti-inflammatory effect | Impact on proliferation and differentiation | Modulation of mitochondrial activity

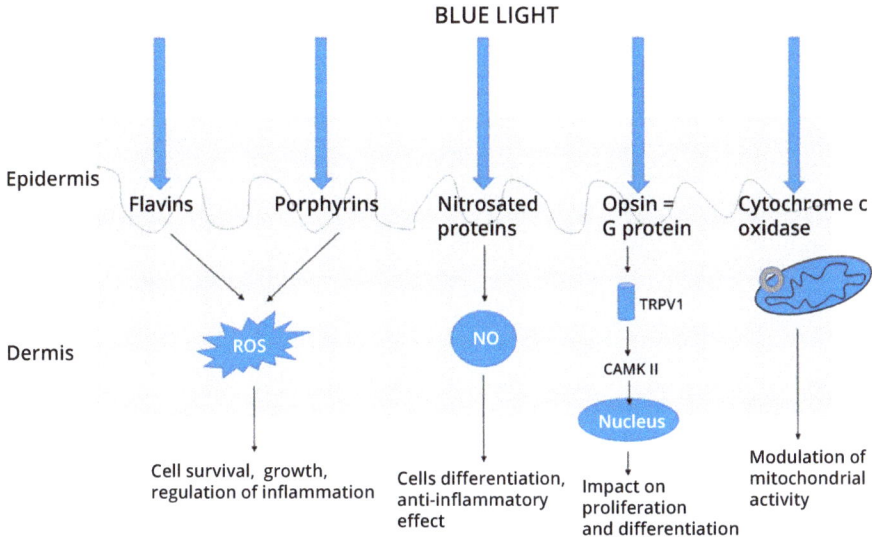

Figure II-6-1. The mechanism of action of blue light (adapted from Sadowska M. et al., 2021)

porphyrins than the latter. KTP radiation causes phototoxic damage to bacteria and, consequently, thermal damage to sebaceous glands. In addition, it is actively absorbed by hemoglobin, which leads to coagulation of dilated capillaries in the area of inflammation, thus reducing its intensity and removing congestion and redness in rashes (Jih M.H., Kimyai-Asadi A., 2007).

No significant side effects of the therapy have been reported. Nonetheless, due to the short-term results, KTP lasers have not gained much popularity in acne therapy.

Pulsed dye lasers (PDL)

PDL generates radiation in the 585–595 nm range, which is actively absorbed by hemoglobin. Initially, these lasers were developed for the correction of vascular disorders. Nowadays, they are also used to treat various conditions in which the vascular component plays a role, including inflammatory skin diseases, particularly acne (Jih M.H., Kimyai-Asadi A., 2007). It is believed that the anti-inflammatory effect of this radiation is achieved by increasing the level of TGF-β as well as through the coagulation of dilated vessels and by reducing the influx of "inflammatory" cells into the lesion area. Thus, not only a reduction in erythema and inflammation but also an improvement in healing is achieved, resulting in marked improvement in post-acne scarring. It has also been recorded that PDL can influence the process of keratinization and comedone formation to some extent. On the other hand, dye lasers do not have a pronounced effect on *C. acnes* or sebum production.

Accordingly, the main indication for their use is the presence of inflammatory rashes.

Infrared lasers
Devices that generate IR radiation can also be used in acne treatment (Jih M.H., Kimyai-Asadi A., 2007), especially:
- Nd:YAG (1064 nm and 1320 nm) (Hügül H. et al., 2023)
- Diode (1450 nm) (Chu G.Y. et al., 2023)

The target chromophore is water, found in all living skin cells, particularly sebum cells. The radiation emitted by IR lasers causes thermal damage to sebocytes, reducing sebum production. Bacteria will also be killed under the influence of such radiation.

Side effects, such as pain during sessions and subsequent redness and swelling, have been noted, but tend to resolve spontaneously. However, their occurrence somewhat reduces the popularity of IR lasers in acne therapy.

Intense pulsed light (IPL)
Unlike lasers that emit strictly defined wavelengths, the lamps used as light sources in IPL devices generate broadband radiation in the 400–1200 nm range. The wavelength spectrum can be altered by special filters, including those designed specifically for acne correction. These filters have bandwidths of 400–600 and 800–1200 nm and are now being actively introduced into practice.

IPL in these spectral ranges exhibits simultaneous effect on various skin chromophores — on *C. acnes* porphyrins and hemoglobin in dilated capillaries (400–600 nm), as well as water in sebocytes (800–1200 nm). The absorption of light energy causes thermal damage to both the targets and the surrounding structures, leading to

ROS formation, TGF-β activation and TNF-α inhibition, vascular coagulation, and sebaceous gland destruction. As a result, the bacteria are eliminated, inflammatory responses are attenuated, and sebum production is reduced (Wu X. et al., 2022).

Several undesirable side effects have been noted after IPL treatment, including transient erythema (in 80% of patients), soreness, swelling, and scaling.

Photodynamic therapy (PDT)

PDT is an "enhanced" version of phototherapy and is one of the main device-based treatments for acne (Li Pomi F. et al., 2024). The chromophores are porphyrins produced by *C. acnes*, but their amounts are usually insufficient for effective treatment. Their quantity can be increased by using special photosensitizers, such as aminolevulinic acid (ALA) or methyl aminolevulinic acid (MLA), which are converted into protoporphyrin IX by interaction with epithelial cells (including sebocytes). ALA also directly stimulates the formation of porphyrins in *C. acnes*.

Further, when this chromophore is exposed to blue and red light, ROS are formed, damaging both bacterial cells and cells of the pilosebaceous complex. In such procedures, lasers, LEDs, fluorescent and arc lamps, incandescent lamps with filters, and IPL devices are used as light sources (Wang D. et al., 2024).

PDT is currently considered one of the most effective device-based treatments for acne. However, due to the accumulation of ALA in epithelial cells, sebocytes and surrounding structures are affected. The side effects of PDT include pain, erythema, edema, burning, crusting, peeling, and hyperpigmentation. This limits the use of classical photosensitizers for the treatment of acne, but newer chlorine-type photosensitizers are now available that selectively accumulate in *C. acnes* and sebocytes, due to which the discomfort and risks associated with the procedures are significantly reduced (Terra Garcia M. et al., 2018).

Photopneumatic therapy

Photopneumatic therapy combines IPL and vacuum (Rajabi-Estarabadi A. et al., 2018; Munavalli G., 2023). The emitting probe draws an area of skin under negative pressure, physically extracting sebum and bringing the sebaceous glands as close as possible to the light source. Vacuum aspiration also lowers blood circulation in the upper layers of the skin, supposedly increasing the procedure's effectiveness. The blue spectrum accounts for photochemical damage to *C. acnes*, and photothermal effects cause damage to sebocytes, resulting in decreased sebum production.

In photopneumatic therapy, undesirable reactions to IPL occur much less frequently and usually take mild forms. Sometimes, petechial hemorrhages are formed under the action of vacuum.

Ultraviolet therapy

Since UV light damages the skin and can provoke malignant cell transformation, in acne treatment, this phototherapy is used only as a last resort.

6.3. Laser therapy and retinoids

There are concerns about using laser therapy while taking isotretinoin, as the drug increases the skin's sensitivity to light and is likely to induce hypertrophic or keloid scarring after trauma. Thus, patients taking isotretinoin are often advised not to subject their skin to surgical or dermatological procedures.

First, non-ablative lasers that emit IR radiation reach deep skin layers, selectively heating the dermis without affecting the epidermis. They are considered safe and effective for skin improvement, requiring minimal recovery time. In many prospective studies, non-ablative lasers have been used to treat mild to moderate acne and post-acne scars. The delicate skin "trauma" after IR laser application is believed to be much less pronounced than after IPL therapy (Sapra S. et al., 2022).

Second, only a few reports describing spontaneous keloid formation after isotretinoin use have been published to date (Bernestein L.J., Geronemus R.G., 1997). One review lists nine studies of combined treatment with oral isotretinoin and laser, including four cohort studies, three case series, and two clinical case studies. Only two publications refer to keloid scarring after combination therapy: in one case, the patient received isotretinoin at a dose of 60 mg/day, and in the other, an unknown dose of the drug was administered (Mysore V. et al., 2019).

A panel of experts from the United States analyzed articles published between 1982 and 2017 to assess the likelihood of complications following phototherapy in patients taking isotretinoin. No strong evidence was found to support the need to delay laser procedures for patients who were currently or in the recent past taking this drug. Shortly thereafter, the American Society for Dermatologic Surgery (ASDS) published a consensus recommendation for physical and surgical interventions during and after isotretinoin therapy. According to the ASDS, the available data does not support the need for delaying chemical peels or non-ablative laser treatments in patients currently or previously taking isotretinoin (Waldman A. et al., 2017).

Moreover, an increasing number of studies suggest that laser procedures can be performed against the background of isotretinoin administration (Prather H.B. et al., 2017).

6.4. Peculiarities of laser application in psoriasis

Psoriasis is one of the most common skin diseases: it affects 2–7% of the world's population and its incidence exhibits a steady upward trend. Psoriasis is characterized as a systemic lesion with dominant manifestations on the skin that tends to remain stable during life or gradually increases in area. Therefore, local treatment of skin foci is prescribed in most cases and is one of the main links in the complex therapy of this disease. As it is a chronic disease, it often requires life-long treatment.

The need for regular application of preparations, which often turns out to be aesthetically unacceptable, significantly reduces patient compliance and, consequently, the effectiveness of prescribed therapy. It is also necessary to note the presence of adverse effects, including systemic reactions, and a wide range of contraindications for the use of most methods and drugs prescribed for topical treatment.

The use of light in psoriasis therapy, first applied in 1925, has been and remains one of the main therapeutic modalities for this pathology. It is natural that the appearance of laser sources contributed to the development and study of their capabilities in treating psoriasis. This is a relatively new direction, which is developing rather slowly due to the "secondary" indications for high-energy lasers that are typically used in esthetic rather than dermatological practice (Zhang P., Wu M.X., 2018).

Advantages of laser treatment of psoriatic skin:
- Affecting psoriatic foci without involving the surrounding skin
- Treatment of pathological foci in any body area (scalp, nails, etc.)
- Minimization of photodamaging and carcinogenic effects and risks of adverse reactions
- No systemic effect on the body
- Comfortable treatment regimen (limited number of treatments, short session time, and long intersession intervals)
- A viable alternative in case of resistance to or refusal of topical therapy
- In most cases, rapid visible positive dynamics and longer remission is achieved
- Combination with local topical agents potentiates the therapeutic effect

The use of lasers opens new therapeutic opportunities. However, lasers allow the achievement of effective results in chronic foci with torpid stable course and limited lesion area (up to 10%), which is currently the main indication for their use. The use of laser radiation in case of a large spread of the process in patients with an unstable course in the progressive stage of the disease is currently considered inappropriate. In these cases, systemic therapy is preferable.

Table II-6-1 summarizes the features of laser therapy for psoriasis, its clinical efficacy, and possible complications.

Excimer laser emitting in the UV spectral range (308 nm) offers very promising results, and has already replaced the previously used UV phototherapy (Ardeleanu V. et al., 2020; Alyoussef A., 2023).

Table II-6-1. Features of laser therapy for psoriasis

	LASER DERMABRASION (FOCI DESTRUCTION)	LOCAL IRRADIATION	SELECTIVE VASCULAR COAGULATION	SPATIALLY MODULATED ABLATION
Device	Er:YAG (2940 nm)	Excimer (308 nm)	PDL (585, 595 nm)	Er:YAG (2940 nm) + SMA
Indica-tions	Single persistent plaques	• Plaque form • Inverse form • Psoriasis of the scalp • Palmoplan-tar form • Nail psoriasis	• Plaque form • Inverse form • Palmoplan-tar form • Nail psoriasis	• Plaque psoriasis • Inverse psoriasis • Scalp psoriasis • Palmoplantar psoriasis
Course	One session, a repeat session is possible after 1–1.5 months	Sessions provided twice a week, aiming for 4–10 or more Cumulative dose should be monitored	At least 5–7 sessions 2–3 weeks apart	At least 1–7 sessions 3–4 weeks apart
Result	Varying degrees of improvement up to complete disappearance of rashes			
Compli-cations	• Dyschromias • Congestive erythema • Wound infection • Scarring	• Formation of blisters, erosions • Hyperpig-mentation	• Formation of blisters and/ or erosions • Pigmenta-tion changes	None noted

Regarding the use of PDL to treat psoriasis, there is an interest-ing hypothesis about its effect. By acting on perivascular nerves, PDL radiation can disrupt the neuroinflammatory processes that cause inflammation in psoriatic foci, leading to prolonged disease relapse. This suggests a potential role for neurogenic inflammation in the development of psoriasis and emphasizes the importance of further research into the interaction between nerves and inflammation in the skin. If this hypothesis proves to be correct, it may open new avenues for the development of targeted psoriasis therapies aimed at modulating neuroinflammatory pathways (Doppegieter M. et al., 2023).

Chapter 7
Laser tattoo removal

The art of tattooing, unique to each historical culture, has existed for many millennia and is now in demand across all age groups, social classes, and professions. Currently, approximately one-third of Americans aged 18–25 and 40% of those aged 26–40 have tattoos. In Germany, 9–12% of the population has tattoos, which are most common (25%) among those aged 18–30.

At the same time, the demand for their removal is also increasing. Available evidence indicates that, about 6% of people request professional tattoo removal 10–15 years after the initial procedure, citing self-esteem issues, as well as changes in social, domestic, and family circumstances. It is postulated that this percentage would likely be higher if consumers were not concerned about the quality of the removal process.

Against the background of well-known methods of tattoo removal such as surgical excision, dermabrasion, and chemical destruction, which lead to the obligatory scar formation, lasers have made it possible to hope for traceless tattoo removal, leaving behind intact skin.

7.1. How do tattoo removal lasers work?

The first reports on laser-assisted tattoo removal appeared in 1965, when L. Goldman presented the results of QS RUBY (694 nm) and Nd:YAG (1064 nm) short-pulsed lasers (Goldman L. et al., 1965). However, the early reports did not arouse due interest, and Argon and CO_2 lasers became the focus of attention. At the time, application of Argon laser (488 and 514 nm) with pulses of 50–200 ms duration resulted in heat propagation from absorbing chromophores (pigment particles) and caused non-selective thermal destruction of tissues, resulting in a high incidence of scarring.

Layer-by-layer tissue removal with a CO_2 laser (10,600 nm), targeting water as the main chromophore, was also shown not to yield satisfactory results, as pigment remained in the tissue after the procedure, and the risks of scarring were high. Attempts to switch from continuous to pulsed mode (50–200 ms), rejection of the idea to remove the dye in one session, reducing the depth of ablation, and stimulation of transepidermal removal through a combination of CO_2 laser with applications of 50% urea, did not lead to a significant reduction in complications. The aesthetic results of treatment remained unpredictable.

These issues persisted until 1983, when R.R. Anderson and J.A. Parrish formulated the principle of selective photothermolysis, resulting in a revolution in the use of laser techniques, including for tattoo removal. The different colors of tattoo ink make them ideal targets for selective photothermolysis. Thus, it became clear that, for effective destruction of dye particles, it is necessary to choose a wavelength that is maximally absorbed by them, minimizing the effect of radiation on endogenous chromophores (oxy- and deoxyhemoglobin, melanin, water). Subsequent investigations further demonstrated that the exposure duration should not exceed the target TRT, preventing the outflow of heat into the surrounding tissues and their damage (Kurniadi I. et al., 2021).

To realize a selective effect on tattoo dye, the pulse duration should be in the ns and ps range, concurring with Goldman's early reports on using short-pulsed lasers (Goldman L. et al., 1965).

Currently, ultrashort-pulsed QS lasers (with powerful pulses of ns to ps duration) are recognized as the "gold standard" for tattoo removal and allow good aesthetic results to be attained without scarring.

However, in practice, devices that emit pulses of light energy in the millisecond range (long-pulsed lasers and IPL) are still used for tattoo removal, which almost always leads to incomplete removal with a significant risk of scarring, including the formation of hypertrophic and keloid scars.

7.2. Tattoo removal lasers

- QS Nd:YAG (1064 nm)
- QS KTP (532 nm)
- PDL (510 nm)
- QS ALEX (755 nm)
- QS RUBY (694 nm)

When QS laser is used, under the influence of a high-energy pulse of ns duration, the dye granules are instantly heated to a temperature above 1000 °C. This leads to a rapid volume expansion with the formation of gaseous pyrolysis products, resulting in a shockwave that fragments the dye particles. In contrast to the initial large-sized granules, which are not amenable to phagocytosis and remain in the skin for prolonged periods, small dye particles can be effectively captured by macrophages and removed through the lymphatic system. The tattoo's color gradually lightens due to a decrease in the dye concentration and the skin is effectively "cleaned" of foreign particles.

Clinically, when a tattoo dye is exposed to QS laser radiation, fragmentation of the tattoo dye is manifested by the instantaneous paling of its color (**Fig. II-7-1**) up to almost complete discoloration (or color change, which occurs more often with pink, red, and beige dyes). White staining may be observed on the skin surface due to the formation of gaseous products. After a few seconds to a few minutes, white staining disappears, and the treated area of the tattoo begins to darken again. This change is caused by mechanical traumatization of small capillaries near the dye granules by the shockwave and formation of specific intradermal hemorrhage in the projection of the tattoo, mimicking its shape. Thus, a focus of aseptic inflammation consisting of macrophage infiltration and intradermal hematoma is formed in the impact zone. Gradually, the focus resolves,

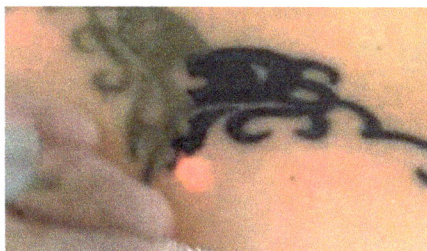

Figure II-7-1. Clinical effect of tattoo dye particle disruption by QS laser

leading to a decrease in the tattoo color intensity compared to the initial clinical picture.

Several sessions are necessary for laser tattoo removal. The number of sessions can vary considerably, depending on the nature of the tattoo and dyes, as well as the adequate selection of radiation parameters, technique, and treatment mode (Hernandez L. et al., 2022).

7.3. Parameters affecting the effectiveness of laser tattoo removal

The success of laser tattoo removal is predetermined by parameters such as:
1. Wavelength
2. Energy density
3. Interval between sessions

The spectral properties of the tattoo dyes determine the choice of wavelength. The absorption spectra of colored pigments are shown in **Fig. II-7-2**.

However, in practice, complex colorants are used, which consist of a mixture of different pigments. Their combination, not each pigment separately, provides the color of the tattoo. Therefore, it is impossible

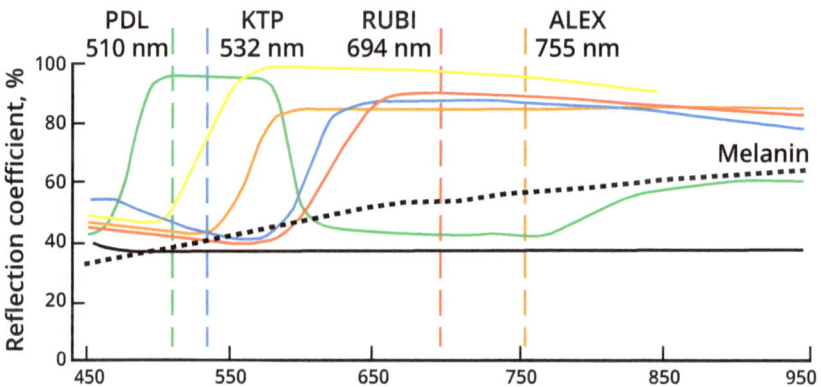

Figure II-7-2. Characteristic absorption spectra of tattoo pigments of basic colors

to classify a tattoo dye as a single pigment, i.e., visually perceived color or cannot uniquely determine its spectral properties, which may vary widely and differ significantly from the data presented above.

Thus, when choosing the wavelength that provides the most effective destruction of the tattoo dye, a test procedure is performed. In the first session, small areas of the tattoo are treated with all types of radiation available.

The optimal laser is the one that has achieved the clinical effect of dye destruction (instant whitening) at the lowest energy density. This type of radiation is selected for further treatment of the remaining untreated part of the tattoo. For polychromatic tattoos, a test procedure is performed for each dye color.

The **energy density** should be sufficient to destroy the tattoo pigment without damaging the skin. If the energy density is suboptimal, the effect on the dye is reduced, which increases the number of required sessions and treatment duration. When excessive energy is applied, not only the target, but also the surrounding tissues are subjected to mechanical destruction, which increases the risk of side effects, including scarring.

The **interval between sessions** is determined by the time required for the resolution of the focus of aseptic inflammation in the the tattoo projection, which depends on many factors, including:

- Individual characteristics of the body (the degree of macrophage response activity, the state of the blood coagulation system which affects the hemorrhage degree, and the intensity of local blood and lymph circulation)
- Features of the tattoo and dye (concentration of dye granules, their size and chemical composition, total tattoo area, its localization)
- Physical parameters of radiation and processing techniques

Factors that increase the area of aseptic inflammation, the concentration of destroyed dye fragments, the degree of tissue damage, and the reduction of the phagocytic activity of macrophages and lymph flow will lengthen the recovery period.

Premature resumption of laser tattoo treatment in conditions of unresolved inflammation dramatically increase the risk of complications because the hematoma shields intact dye granules. Its destruction (obtaining the clinical effect in the form of pale tattoo coloring) requires a significant increase in energy density, increasing the degree of traumatization of the surrounding tissues. Moreover, untimely subsequent session will not lead to increased efficiency, because it will affect macrophages containing phagocytized microparticles of previously destroyed dye that have not yet been removed from the focus of inflammation.

In practice, it is difficult to consider all factors and calculate a sufficient time interval in each specific case, so most specialists rely on the average timeframe, which is about two months. In our practice, the time needed for the resolution of aseptic inflammation varies considerably from the average values, as some patients need less while others require much more time to recover. The possibility of shortening the interval in some patients allows us to reduce the treatment course duration, while greater intervals help avoid probable complications.

The following criteria are used to determine the optimal timeframe for the next tattoo removal session:

- Pale coloration of the tattoo compared to the state before the previous session.
- Achievement of dye destruction in the form of pallor at the same energy density parameters as in the previous session. If such clinical effect is achieved, but is weak (due to a decrease in dye concentration), the energy density can be increased by 1–2 scale points. If the parameters used in the previous session are not clinically effective, it is necessary to stop the treatment and postpone the session for two weeks with a re-evaluation of the criteria for resolution of the aseptic inflammation focus.

7.4. Factors that complicate laser tattoo removal

The **photochemical effect** is characterized by the transformation of the chemical composition of the dye under the influence of laser radiation, which externally manifests as a change in the tattoo color. Along with the chemical composition, the spectral properties of the pigment change, and consequently, its sensitivity to the selected type of laser. As a rule, the photochemical effect is characteristic of dyes containing metals (iron, titanium, etc.); under the influence of radiation, their oxides are transformed from one type to another. Photochemical reaction typically manifests in red, pink, beige, and white dyes, which change their color to grayish–green or black when treated with laser.

The possibility of photochemical effects should be considered, and the patient should be warned of this risk in advance. To avoid aesthetically unacceptable results, the smallest and most inconspicuous area of the tattoo should be treated first.

Photochemical reactions to laser exposure can also be observed in black and blue dyes. As a rule, they are less noticeable and are expressed in the darkening of the dye or change of its shade. Sometimes, such changes develop gradually, from one session to the next, gaining clarity only after 4–5 sessions, when the concentration of newly formed pigment becomes high enough. As the tattoo "freezes" at this point, in the subsequent sessions, there is no significant change in dye intensity under the influence of laser.

A typical mistake, in this case, is to increase the energy density with a decrease in the diameter of the light spot, as this increases the impact on the epidermis and the superficial layer of the dermis, where there is little dye — the efficiency of destruction does not increase, and the risk of skin damage with subsequent scarring increases. In such cases, it is necessary to repeat the test procedure by selecting another laser. If it is possible to find an effective radiation, treatment should be continued, and a non-selective method with ablative lasers (Er:YAG, CO_2) should be adopted otherwise.

Multilayered tattoos are obtained by superimposing a new drawing on the previous one. In this area there are two (or more) types of dyes that respond differently to the effects of laser radiation: one absorbs the selected wavelength well, while the other is less responsive or does not absorb radiation of this energy at all. During the laser session, the old pattern may appear. It is often necessary to sequentially remove one dye at the time, while changing laser type as needed. Therefore, removal of overlapped tattoos, as a rule, requires a significantly longer treatment course.

It should also be noted that repeated dye injection to the same site increases the degree of traumatization and leads to microscar formation. When the dye is removed, the changed skin structure in the projection of the former tattoo may visually differ from the surrounding normal skin, taking on a whitish tint. The patient should be warned about this possibility before treatment.

3D tattoos are produced by using a very high concentration of dye in a single layer, due to which the tattoo appears to be raised above the level of the surrounding skin. The difficulty of removing such tattoos stems from the fact that the distance between the dye particles is very small, so the mechanical waves coming from closely located chromophores meet each other and sum up, resulting in a sharp increase in their amplitude which is sufficient to destroy the surrounding tissue.

Reduction of energy density parameters does not result in the desired clinical effect of dye destruction. To reduce the risk of scarring, it is necessary to reduce the chromophore concentration before proceeding with selective tattoo removal. For this purpose, a non-selective method with the help of ablative lasers (CO_2, Er:YAG) should be performed first, due to the vaporization of superficial skin layers together with excess pigment. It is possible to continue tattoo removal with QS lasers after full skin recovery (in about one month).

Tattoos complicated by skin deformation due to scarring require more time for removal. The existing scarring disturbances of the skin structure in the tattoo projection hinder the elimination of destroyed dye particles by macrophages from the treatment zone. Therefore, the resolution of the focus of aseptic inflammation after laser treatment is generally slower, and the intervals between sessions are lengthened.

In addition, with fresh (up to 12 months old) hypertrophic and keloid scars, there is a risk of dye exposure to the laser radiation, which may provoke scar tissue growth. Therefore, such tattoos require a special approach, whereby either the correction of the scar should precede dye removal, or it is necessary to use combined exposure methods, affecting both the tattoo dye and scar tissue. In our practice, we combine selective removal of tattoo pigment by QS lasers with SMA module in one session, which optimizes dye elimination and the intersession interval duration, while having a corrective effect on the scar.

7.5. Factors limiting laser tattoo removal

The **insensitivity of tattoo dyes** to the types of laser radiation used excludes the possibility of their fragmentation and removal by lymphatic flow. In this case, they can be removed only by non-selective methods, such as skin ablation with CO_2 or Er:YAG laser.

Traumatic tattoos are impregnations of various kinds of particles (dirt, asphalt, gunpowder, chemicals, etc.) that cannot be fragmented, or their destruction may be accompanied by an explosion or toxic reaction. Such tattoos should thus be removed with ablative lasers.

Tattoos may be complicated by allergic reaction to the dye characterized by granulomatous inflammation. As a result, the tissues in the tattoo projection are thickened, and the relief becomes lumpy and raised. Such a reaction is most frequently observed in red dyes. Selective laser dye destruction in the presence of allergic granuloma should not be attempted. There is a great danger of the spread of allergic reactions beyond the site of its primary manifestation with the generalization of the process because the removal of dye particles occurs via lymphatic ducts.

Accordingly, dye and granuloma removal should be performed simultaneously by laser ablation, and some specialists believe that only surgical excision is advised in such cases. In the available literature, two cases of allergic reactions to red-ink tattoos after treatment with CO_2 laser are described. In one of the patients, generalized hypersensitivity reaction appeared after the fifth procedure, which the authors attributed to incomplete removal of allergenic particles during the tattoo treatment (Meesters A.A. et al., 2016). Willardson H.B. et al. (2017) described four cases of allergic reactions encountered in their practice, one of which was particularly challenging. A 46-year-old female patient presented with urticaria, erythema, and pruritus following multiple Nd:YAG tattoo removal attempts. The systemic allergic reaction proved resistant to increasing doses of antihistamines and corticosteroids. As a result, the tattoo had to be surgically removed. When the excised tissue was analyzed by scanning electron microscopy (SEM) and energy dispersive X-ray analysis (EDXA), a high level of titanium dioxide was found. Two weeks after tattoo excision, the urticaria resolved without the use of drug therapy. This case demonstrated a strong association of a common allergic reaction with titanium dioxide in tattoo pigments following laser tattoo removal.

No assurance of the dye's safety when it breaks down can be presently given. The demand for uniform regulation of tattoo ink ingredients in Europe has led to the need for analytical methods suitable for identifying banned compounds. Poor solubility and lack of volatility are common problems associated with most pigments and polymers used in tattoo inks. By pyrolytic-gas chromatography/mass spectrometry, 28 commercially available and most frequently used tattoo inks, as well and 18 homemade pigment mixtures were investigated (Schreiver I. et al., 2016).

Based on the obtained data, models were created to predict the degradation of pigments when tattoos are exposed to laser irradiation, sunlight, or other factors. This makes it possible to assess the risks to consumers associated with the toxic effects of pigment degradation products and to identify more or less harmful pigments for this application.

7.6. Skincare after laser tattoo removal

If treatment based on the optimal choice of laser radiation and adequately selected energy density does not damage the skin surface, the patient should be advised to avoid traumatizing this area, refrain from UV exposure for two weeks after the treatment, and use high-grade sunscreen filters locally to prevent dyschromic disorders.

If crusts and blisters form due to improper selection of radiation parameters and treatment technique, reparative means (creams with dexpanthenol) and hydrogel dressings are recommended. Careful wound management will be crucial for obtaining a good aesthetic effect of tattoo removal.

7.7. Complications of laser tattoo removal

When removing tattoos using QS lasers, complications are possible and usually involve scarring and dyschromia of the skin in the treatment area. They can be caused by incorrectly selecting the physical parameters of radiation and treatment technique for the case characteristics (high phototype, tendency to pathological scarring), as well as by patient's non-compliance with the recommendations.

7.8. What has been done to improve laser tattoo removal?

Change of the QS pulse mode. Instead of a single pulse (duration of the order of tens of nanoseconds), typical for classical lasers with modulated QS, a series of ns-long pulses with a millisecond sequence is used. The power of each pulse in the series is sufficient to destroy the dye in a thin tattoo layer. Each subsequent pulse in a series penetrates progressively deeper, allowing fragments of the pigment to reach the full depth of its occurrence in the tattoo, increasing each session's effectiveness. At the same time, the damage to the surrounding tissues is reduced because a thin layer of dye can be destroyed at a lower energy density. When using a classical QS laser, when a single pulse is applied, the energy density for effective dye destruction across the entire tattoo thickness must be much higher, which increases the traumatization of the surrounding tissues and the risk of complications. Reduced power, on the other hand, decreases efficiency, necessitating a greater number of tattoo removal procedures.

Multiple consecutive tattoo passes in a single session:
- R20 method: Typically, 3–4 passes are performed, with an interval of 20 min (after resolution of whitening of treated tissues due to micro-cavitation bubble formation). This approach is not widely used in practice because the time interval between passes significantly lengthens the procedure.
- R0 method (optimized R20): This approach involves the use of patches with perfluorodecalin, which rapidly removes whitening

by absorbing gaseous pyrolysis products. No time interval between passes is required, which makes the method more convenient for practical use.

Perfluorodecalin patches. One of the most popular methods for improving laser tattoo removal results is the use of the drug perfluorodecalin. It is an inert colorless fluorocarbon liquid, which quickly eliminates whitening due to the absorption of gaseous products formed during the destruction of tattoo pigments.

Perfluorodecalin reduces optical scattering near the skin surface so that the increased flux density reaches deeply situated pigment particles. Even more practical and effective is the use of a patch with perfluorodecalin, as it prevents the evaporation of liquid perfluorodecalin and increases the thermal protection of the epidermis. This effect is achieved because the direct contact between the skin, silicone, and perfluorodecalin allows a more efficient heat dissipation from the skin surface. It is believed that perfluorodecalin allows practitioners to perform several passes in one procedure, as well as improves patient tolerance and reduces the incidence of adverse events associated with epidermal damage, such as erythema and edema (Reddy K.K. et al., 2013).

Combined protocols based on ablative techniques and selective laser tattoo dye removal:

- Sequential application of ablative treatment for removing the superficial skin with pigment and — after recovery — selective laser dye removal.
- The combination of selective dye destruction with fractional ablative methods and SMA increases the efficiency of dye destruction, reduces the inter-session interval due to the activation of macrophage response, and minimizes the probability of negative side effects.

Picosecond lasers. Lasers emitting radiation of 755, 785, 532 and 1064 nm wavelength are currently on the market. The pulse duration varies from 375 to 750 ps.

Evidence shows that picosecond lasers are relatively more effective and safer for tattoo removal than their nanosecond counterparts

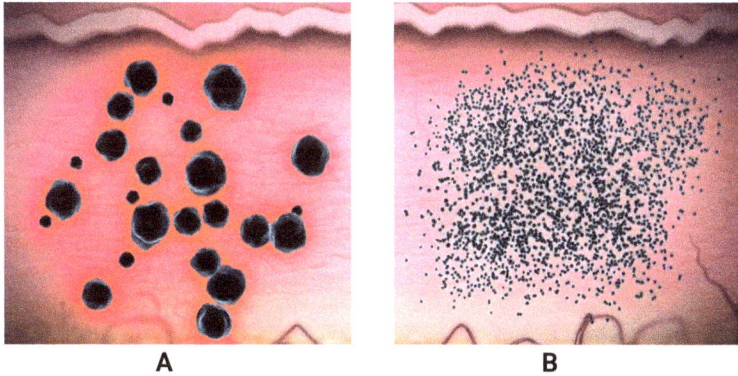

Figure II-7-3. Tattoo dye fragmentation by nano- and picosecond laser

(Leu F.J. et al., 2022). This is likely because picosecond lasers fragment the pigment into smaller particles that are more easily removed from the tissue (**Fig. II-7-3**).

Successful removal of red and black professional tattoos in patients with Fitzpatrick skin type VI using 532-nm ps Nd:YAG laser was also reported in literature (Friedman D.J., 2016).

Laser tattoo removal methods have firmly entered the skin-care practice and are popular among clients. At present, QS lasers, capable of effectively destroying tattoo components while protecting the skin from unwanted trauma, demonstrate great efficiency in achieving optimal aesthetic results. Highly qualified specialists, the right choice of radiation type and its parameters, and the optimal mode and treatment technique can yield predictable good aesthetic outcomes. However, the significant treatment duration and the high prevalence of complex clinical cases, in which it was not possible to achieve complete dye removal, highlight the need for new solutions. Modern trends indicate that the research focus should be on active, scientifically and practically justified improvements of existing methods, development of new devices, and optimization of pigment composition used for tattooing.

More information on tattoo pigment removal methods can be found in the *Tattoos and Permanent Makeup: Skin Care and Removal in Cosmetic Dermatology and Skincare Practice* book.

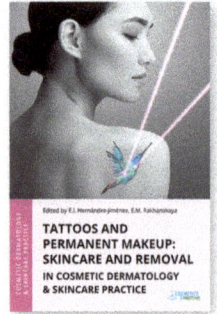

Chapter 8
Light-based epilation

The hair structure includes many components, with the hair shaft as the only visible part. The shaft is produced in the hair follicle, hidden deep in the skin. The follicle is the main target of hair removal. However, regardless of the hair removal method, the hair shaft is an energy conductor to the follicle.

The hair removal outcome is related to the hair growth phase in which the follicle is affected, whereby three stages are distinguished:

1. **Anagen (growth stage):** The hair follicle can be reached only in the anagen. In this stage, the hair shaft and the follicle are closely connected.
2. **Catagen (transitional stage):** The hair follicle at this stage is characterized by several morphological features. The main one is that the epithelial sheath still exists, which indicates slow hair shaft growth.
3. **Telogen (resting period):** The hair shaft does not grow and eventually falls out; the hair follicle is characterized by a keratinized, thickened root with remnants of pigment granules.

The number of hairs in the anagen stage is variable and depends on its localization on the body. On average, 80–88% of the scalp's hair is in the anagen, 1% in the catagen, and 20% in the telogen stage. The growth cycles of neighboring hairs are not synchronous, so young and old hairs are simultaneously present in all skin areas. The eyebrow and ear canal areas have only 15% of hair in anagen, the chin area 70%, the upper lip 65%, and the legs and bikini line 30%. The anagen duration also varies:

- 4–8 weeks on eyebrows and ears
- 10–12 months on the chin
- Up to 4 months on legs, bikini, and upper lip
- Up to 8 years on the head

The first and foremost law of hair removal states that, for hair growth to cease, the hair follicle must be destroyed during the anagen stage.

8.1. How do laser and photoepilation work?

Depending on the light source, light-based epilation is subdivided into:
1. **Laser hair removal (laser epilation)** by laser devices
2. **Photoepilation** by IPL devices

The targets of light-based epilation are the hair-producing keratinocytes (in the dermal papilla) and the stem cells that give rise to these keratinocytes (in the *bulge*) (**Fig. II-8-1**). Neither of these has a chromophore that light energy can selectively act upon (at least none has been found to date).

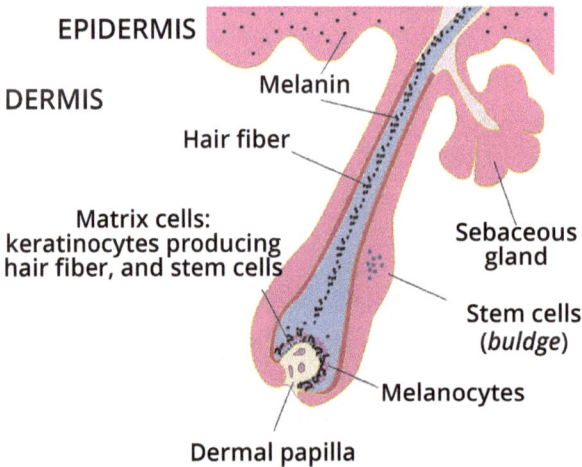

Figure II-8-1. The matrix contains fast-dividing keratinocytes that produce the hair shaft. Melanocytes are located among the keratinocytes in the lower part of the hair follicle. Stem cells localized in the bulge area migrate to the dermal papilla to differentiate into keratinocytes

Therefore, melanocytes, which produce melanin, and dead hair shaft cells filled with melanin are used to generate destructive heat. When melanin absorbs red and IR light, it enters an excited state, and then gives off energy in the form of heat, which primarily damages the melanocytes and nearby living cells. Heat spreads along the hair shaft to the follicular epithelium and damages it. Since the skin has a shorter TRT than the hair, its temperature increase will always be significantly lower due to the rapid heat dissipation. The light pulse duration is determined by the TRT.

Accordingly, extended selective photothermolysis is realized herein: the target is affected by secondary heat, and there is a distance between the heat generator and the primary target (Altshuler G.B. et al., 2001; Ross E.V., 2001).

Engineers and epilation specialists are yet to reach a consensus regarding the light energy parameters:

1. On the one hand, energy must be **sufficient** not just to overcome the distance between melanocytes and stem cells but to destroy stem cells thermally.
2. On the other hand, it must be **insufficient** for causing damage the interfollicular epidermis and adjacent dermis.

The evolution of light-based epilation technology reflects the search for a solution to this issue, which most directly relates to the efficacy/safety aspects of the procedure and its tolerability by the client (Gold M.H. et al., 2023).

Notably, the exact mechanism of hair growth disruption during light-based epilation remains unknown. Unlike household hair removal methods, the effect of photoepilation is prolonged; that is, hair growth continues to be disturbed, and the number of hairs continues to decrease after treatment is completed. Several hypotheses have been proposed:

1. Heat causes coagulation of the vessels that feed the hair follicle, which leads to gradual follicle atrophy and hair growth cessation.
2. Heat triggers the programmed death of the follicular epithelium cells, which leads to atrophy of the follicle.
3. The regulation of hair growth phases is disturbed due to the disruption of interactions between follicle growth cells.

8.2. Important features of hair and skin during epilation

Melanin, the target chromophore in hair removal, is found in hair and skin, so we need to damage the former without affecting the latter. In this regard, the color of the hair and skin in light-based epilation is essential.

Color depends on many factors, the most important of which are genetic and endocrine. The wide range of hair color — from the lightest to black — is mainly due to two pigments: black–brown eumelanin and yellow–red pheomelanin, which differ in granule size. Variants depend on the quantitative ratio of these pigments, while the change in hair color during life is due to the dynamics of the general endocrine background. Both eumelanin and pheomelanin are synthesized in melanocytes located in the hair follicle above the papilla. Melanocytes produce pigment only during the anagen phase of hair growth. To determine the correct principles of laser hair removal, it is important to understand that black, blond, red, and gray hair may respond differently to the light pulse.

Melanin (eumelanin and pheomelanin) is also found in the skin. Different people's skin will differ in its ability to produce melanin, in the distribution of melanocytes, and in its blood supply. The lighter the skin and the less melanin it contains, the less "competitive" its absorption of laser energy. At the same time, people with darker skin phototypes have an excess of melanin. The same problem exists in people with a tan. Because of this, the skin can get very hot, increasing the risk of burns, while hair follicles and hair shafts "under-receive" the required amount of laser radiation and are not destroyed. As a result, the incidence of adverse reactions during laser hair removal is much greater in dark-skinned relative to light-skinned patients. Specialists are trying to get around this limitation by experimenting with different wavelengths, energy density, and other parameters (Fayne R.A. et al., 2018).

Thomas Fitzpatrick classified skin types based on the skin's ability to respond to UV radiation (**Table II-8-1**). The same classification is used to predict photoepilation outcome and select the radiation source.

Table II-8-1. Skin phototypes, according to Fitzpatrick

PHOTOTYPE	DESCRIPTION
I	Never tan, always burn (usually excessively white skin, blond hair, blue/green eyes)
II	Sometimes tan, but more often burn (fair skin, blond or brown hair, green/brown eyes)
III	Often tan, sometimes burn (medium skin, brown hair, brown eyes)
IV	Always tan, never burn (olive skin, dark hair, dark eyes)
V	Never burn (dark brown skin, black hair, black eyes)
VI	Never burn (dark brown to black skin, black hair, black eyes)

Currently, laser hair removal can be performed on people with any skin and hair color, so it is important to select the appropriate radiation parameters (Dorgham N.A., Dorgham D.A., 2020). However, on average, treatment in patients with black and brown hair achieves better effects than in those with red, blond, or gray hair. In addition, the longer the wavelength used, the less effective epilation is in those with light-colored hair, because long-wave radiation is poorly absorbed by melanin, which is already scarce in this hair type. In addition, in patients with light-colored hair, temporary hair reduction (for up to three months) is typically achieved, whereas most patients with brown and black hair have a growth delay of 2–6 months after a single session.

Human skin also varies in the epidermis thickness and hair depth. In men, the epidermis is usually thicker, the skin produces more fat, and the follicles are deeper (**Fig. II-8-2**). These skin characteristics should be considered when epilating transsexual men who have changed their gender to female.

A good response to laser hair removal occurs when the target hair contains chromophores in high concentration. Accordingly, terminal (long, dense) hairs are the best candidates for laser hair removal. At the same time, vellus (short, thin, light-colored) hair contains little melanin. Consequently, it absorbs light energy poorly and is inadequately destroyed. This outcome is expected when treating areas such as the upper lip, where there is little chromophore, and the hair is

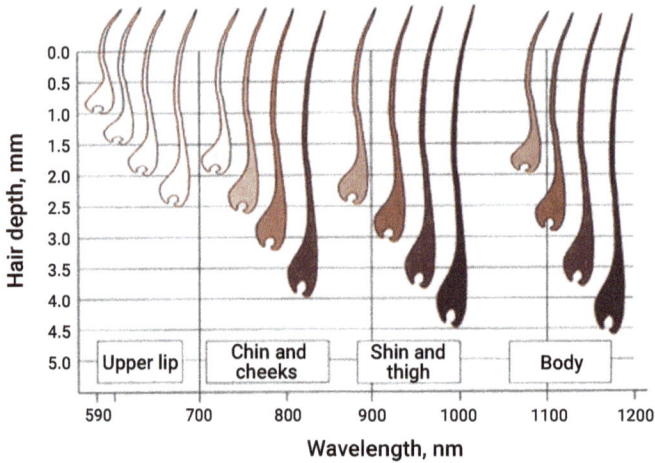

Figure II-8-2. Radiation wavelength selection depending on hair color, location, and depth

quite "delicate." As far as shaft thickness is concerned, epilation of hair with a diameter below 30 μm is not particularly effective.

8.3. Important parameters of laser and IPL devices for hair removal

Modern devices for light-based and laser hair removal are equipped with a control unit that allows practitioners to select the light exposure parameters based on the skin phototype and patient characteristics (the threshold of sensitivity in particular). They should be selected in the following order:

1. Light spot size (mm)
2. Pulse duration (ms)
3. Energy flux density (J/cm²)

As for the wavelength, in monochrome laser devices, it is fixed, while in IPL systems, a range of wavelengths (e.g., 560–1200 nm or 650–1200 nm) is set. In hair removal, the **melanin window** — a spectral range in which it makes sense to work if we want to affect melanin and minimize the impact on other chromophores — is important.

The melanin window includes radiation emitted by RUBY (694 nm), ALEX (755 nm), Diode (800–810 nm), and Nd:YAG (1064 nm) lasers, as well as IPL devices. All these radiation emitters, except the RUBY laser, are currently used in specific devices for light-based epilation, which indicates that the "best" light source does not exist, and the presented examples are more or less comparable in their effectiveness.

By increasing the radiation power and shortening the pulse duration, the zone of boundary heating can be reduced, preventing thermal damage (burns) to the adjacent skin.

Various substances transparent to the laser beam and possessing high thermal conductivity (ice, gels, artificial sapphire) are currently used for skin cooling during the session. Colling allows for a high exposure selectivity and significantly reduces the likelihood of thermal damage to the skin. However, it is not possible to completely eliminate the risk of skin burns. The risk increases with an increase in:

- Melanin in the skin surrounding the follicle
- Hair density and hair shaft thickness
- Pulse energy and radiation power
- Pulse duration

In each specific case, it is necessary to select the radiation energy and pulse duration based on the individual characteristics of the patient's skin and hair. At the same time, the success of epilation is completely determined by the choice of the radiation source, its technical characteristics, its mode of operation, and cooling systems.

8.4. Laser and photoepilation devices

8.4.1. Lasers

A high-density laser beam can produce a significant local thermal effect, accompanied by reactive coagulation of the follicular zone, vaporization, and carbonization (charring) of the tissue surrounding the follicle. Simply put, the follicle is burned, dried, and charred. The computer software imbedded in the laser systems allows for precisely targeted selective action so that all these effects take place only in the area surrounding the hair follicle. In addition to thermal effects, the light produces other effects (photoelectric, biostimulating, etc.), but thermal effects predominate when the radiation source power is high.

Destruction of the hair follicle with a laser beam is possible only if there is a chromophore in the beam's path which absorbs radiation in the red range (it is the radiation that penetrates the skin the deepest) and is concentrated mainly in the hair. Otherwise, spontaneous deactivation of the beam occurs (in other words, it is simply scattered). In the skin, the chromophore is melanin, and its content in the hair shaft is also very high. Instead of melanin, practitioners can choose some exogenous chromophore (dye) that will selectively color the hair.

RUBY, ALEX, Diode, and Nd:YAG lasers emit the most suitable radiation for hair removal.

RUBY was the first laser to appear on the hair removal market. It emits red light of 694 nm wavelength in 3-ms pulses, providing an energy flow of up to 40–60 J/cm^2. The pulse repetition rate is 1 Hz, so it is a relatively slow-acting laser. Since the target is exclusively the hair melanin (hemoglobin absorbs weakly at this wavelength), the laser cannot be used on tanned skin because its energy will be dissipated, and due to a high risk of skin damage. In addition, it does not "recognize" light-colored hair. The effectiveness of RUBY epilation is the highest in phototypes I–II with dark hair. It is unsuitable for the removal of light and red hair and hair on tanned skin or phototypes IV–V. However, even in individuals with dark hair, sometimes epilation does not have the desired effect. At the same time, RUBY is the most well-tested type of laser and is most widely used in clinical trials involving light-based hair removal. Interestingly, after RUBY epilation, the follicle does not die but goes into catagen and telogen phases. That is, cessation of hair growth is achieved by the disruption of the normal growth cycle.

ALEX emits radiation of 755 nm wavelength, resulting in minimal hemoglobin absorption and strong melanin absorption. Procedures are performed with targeted manipulators with a radiation beam of 10–30 mm diameter (Piccolo D. et al., 2023). With the 10–20 J/cm^2

energy density, pulse duration of 15–30 ms and 5 Hz pulse frequency, it is five times faster than RUBY.

More than 95% of ALEX radiation is absorbed by melanin. The absorbed energy is transformed into heat, causing "burning" of the hair shaft and thermal destruction of the hair follicle and its feeding vessel. If the hair is in the anagen stage, when there is a close connection between the feeding vessel and the sprouting zone, hair growth is not observed after the session. Within a few weeks after the treatment, the coagulated hair root falls out. Procedures are carried out every 4–8 weeks depending on the epilation area. With each subsequent session, the number of hairs within the treated area decreases, and the rate of their growth slows down. To achieve permanent hair removal at least five procedures are recommended and the treatment should be repeated 2–3 times after 12 months to remove the remaining hairs.

Unfortunately, due to the competitive absorption of this laser radiation by melanin of the interfollicular epidermis, the procedure can only be performed on skin of phototype I–IV and with mandatory cooling to prevent burns and dyschromia. This procedure is still considered the "gold standard" for the epilation of dark hair on light skin.

Nd:YAG epilation is based on the homogeneous absorption of light by oxy-, deoxyhemoglobin, and various protein structures, which are consequently heated, causing coagulation of the delivery vessel and destruction of highly differentiated cells and germinative zones of the hair follicle. Due to the very low absorption capacity of melanin at this wavelength (about 10%), the competition between skin and hair pigment is eliminated. That is why when using neodymium laser on light-colored hair, hair shaft is not burned and the likelihood of complications in the form of dyschromia is much lower than when the ALEX laser is used. Today, Nd:YAG is the device of choice for working with dark skin phototypes and light hair. Due to the uniform absorption of radiation at 1064 nm by tissues, the procedure is more painful compared to those based on ALEX laser, and is thus only suitable for some patients. The effectiveness of epilation with this type of laser is quite low: after one session, 40% of hair grows after a month, and the number doubles after three months. Therefore, especially when working with light-colored hair, the amount of hair begins to decrease only after the third session. Accordingly, at least eight treatments are required.

Currently, the laser of choice in patients with dark phototypes and tanned skin is long-pulsed 1064-nm Nd:YAG, as its radiation is less absorbed by melanin, but the effectiveness of epilation will be less pronounced. At the same time, Nd:YAG is more effective than IPL. The 810-nm Diode laser has also been shown to be more effective for epilation in people with dark skin phototypes compared to the 755-nm ALEX laser because its radiation penetrates deeper into the dermis (**Table II-8-2**).

Table II-8-2. Epilation lasers: ALEX, Nd:YAG, and hybrid Diode

ALEX (755 nm) "The gold standard" for dark hair removal on light skin (phototypes I–III)	HYBRID DIODE LASER (755/810 nm)
The primary target is melanin	The primary target is melanin
Cannot be used in phototypes above IV due to the risk of burning the perifollicular epidermis	Can be adapted to work with all phototypes
Ineffective for light-colored hair	Removes light and fine hair
Penetrates up to 3 mm deep, which is sometimes not enough	Deeper penetration into the skin

ND:YAG (1064 nm) "Gold standard" for hair removal on skin phototypes III–IV	HYBRID DIODE LASER (810/1064 nm)
The primary target is oxyhemoglobin	The main targets are melanin and oxyhemoglobin
Effective for epilation of light-colored hair with low melanin content Poorly removes dark hair	Removes both dark and light-colored hairs
Penetrates the entire depth of the dermis, destroying deep follicles	Destroys both deep and superficial follicles
Painful procedure	Less painful procedure

ALEX/Nd:YAG delivers a combination of two wavelengths — 755/1064 nm — allowing practitioners to use much lower (2–3 times) energy densities of laser radiation, and epilation with such combined radiation is safer.

Radiation at 755 nm is absorbed by the melanin in hair, causing its coagulation, but without significant damage to the growth zone and feeding vessels, because the density of the supplied energy is not high enough. With the simultaneous use of 755 and 1064 nm wavelengths, homogeneous photothermolysis is added to selective absorption of light energy by coagulated tissues. Thus, Nd:YAG targets the ALEX-prepared tissue. Because the coagulated hair shaft has a strong broad-spectrum absorption coefficient, the flash energy density of the neodymium laser can be significantly lower than when it is applied alone.

Diode laser generates invisible light of 800–810 nm wavelength in the near-IR part of the spectrum, i.e., coinciding with the melanin absorption peak. The pulse duration is 5 to 30 ms, the frequency is 1 Hz, and the energy flux on tissue is 10–40 J/cm² in a laser spot with a 9 mm diameter. Like RUBY, a diode-based laser cannot effectively epilate light-colored and red hair, or hair on tanned skin. Technical adaptations of Diode lasers for hair removal are proceeding in different directions. For example, laser radiation is combined with vacuum action in the tip of the LightSheer DUET device (Lumenis, USA). The tip is shaped like a dome and is connected to a vacuum pump, which, when turned on, creates negative pressure, and the skin is lifted, bringing it closer to the radiating elements. As a result:

- The distance between the follicles and the transmitter is reduced.
- The epidermis is stretched, and the density of melanin in it consequently decreases; therefore, the skin adjacent to the follicle is heated to a lesser extent, and the risk of thermal damage to it decreases.
- Partial constriction of blood vessels occurs, and hemoglobin concentration in the affected area decreases.
- Light scattering is reduced due to the larger spot size and the presence of reflective surfaces (the tip's inner surface has a special coating).

- Pain is reduced: due to the distracting effect of negative pressure on tactile receptors, the neurosynaptic "switch" in the spinal cord that transmits the pain impulse to the brain is blocked (according to the "gateway" theory of pain).

Thus, in the skin area located under the tip, when the vacuum pump is turned on, there is a significant reduction in the number of competitive chromophores due to a decrease in melanin density and hemoglobin concentration. This fact, along with the proximity of follicles to the transmitter, allows the energy flow to be reduced to about 12 J/cm^2 instead of the usual 30–40 J/cm^2, which guarantees a high level of safety and provides maximal efficiency (hair is removed permanently after 3–4 sessions). At the same time, the spot size is large enough, which is convenient for treating large body areas. This means that less time is required for the procedure (on average, the treatment duration is reduced by 60%). The resulting anesthetic effect makes the procedure comfortable and easily tolerated without local anesthesia.

Another very promising trend involves the use of **hybrid Diode lasers**, which are based on a combination of diodes emitting at different wavelengths (see **Table II-8-2**). In addition to good performance and safety, Diode lasers have other important advantages:
- Convenient and lightweight probe to the multifunctional platform instead of big traditional laser devices
- The spot size is larger than for traditional lasers: 12 × 26 mm (3 cm^2)
- Optimized pulse modes in terms of duration, frequency, and power
- Efficient and comfortable cooling system at maximum energy and all ambient temperatures

8.4.2. IPL

Photoepilation is performed using a non-monochromatic lamp emitting in a broad spectral range, i.e., within the 500–1200 nm wavelength span, which overlaps with the area of high absorption by melanin. Unlike lasers, the lamp projects a 4.5-cm^2 square-shaped spot onto the skin. A light flux of 35–55 J/cm^2 is provided by a series of up to five consecutive pulses of 2–5 ms duration. The effect is due to photo-thermal follicle death, and the intervals between pulses allow the skin to cool down when exposed to high energies (Kang C.N. et al., 2021).

8.5. Hormonal impact on laser epilation and photoepilation outcome

The results of laser hair removal can be affected by various hor-monal diseases and conditions of the body, such as polycystic ovary syndrome, thyroid dysfunction, adrenal hyperplasia, hyperprolac-tinemia, and others. Suppose the specialist suspects that the patient has a hormonal pathology. In that case, the procedure should be post-poned and the patient should be referred to a general practitioner, gynecologist, endocrinologist, or other specialist for examination.

8.5.1. Hirsutism and hypertrichosis

Hirsutism is the excessive growth of thick or dark hair in women on areas of the body that are more typical for males (e.g., mustache, beard, hair on the central chest, shoulders, lower abdomen, back, in-ner thighs). The intensity of hair growth that is considered excessive can vary according to ethnicity and cultural beliefs. Hypertrichosis is another condition in which there is an increase in the amount of hair on any part of the body. Hypertrichosis can be generalized or localized.

In some women with a mild degree of hirsutism or hypertrichosis, hormonal disorders may be present, including Cushing's syndrome, various tumors, etc. Sometimes there is also idiopathic hirsutism — excessive hair without an apparent cause. Diagnosis is reached by exclusion, whereby doctors suspect this condition when all other pos-sible causes of the disease have been ruled out. In any case, this con-dition requires a qualified, comprehensive evaluation. Establishing the cause of hirsutism and hypertrichosis followed by the treatment of the underlying endocrine disorder is important for the proper man-agement of these patients, especially women. Oral contraceptives sup-press the production of luteinizing and follicle-stimulating hormones, resulting in decreased androgen production in the ovaries and adrenal glands. Low androgenic progestins are preferred because they antagonize 5α-reductase and androgen receptors. Patients with untreated hormonal conditions may have an uneven or poor response to laser hair removal and, on average, require a greater number of sessions than patients with normal hormone levels (Lee C.M., 2018).

8.5.2. Hyperprolactinemia

In pregnancy, there is an increase in prolactin levels: this condition has a melanocyte-stimulating effect. In this case, it is essential to appreciate that all light-based treatment methods will be ineffective.

Hyperprolactinemia is a very important factor in poor hair response to laser treatment. Even if patients are treated, hair removal will not work correctly until the hyperprolactinemia is controlled. In these patients, prolactin levels are in the 30–90 ng/dL range and these values indicate that, regardless of wavelength choice and device capabilities, acceptable results will not be achieved. There is also evidence of reduced hair response to laser hair removal in women with polycystic ovary syndrome, which is often associated with hyperprolactinemia (Nabi N. et al., 2022).

Hyperprolactinemic conditions not only cause increased melanocyte-stimulating hormone activity, but also affect the reactivation of stem progenitor cells in the hair follicle and *bulge* area. Hirsutism in hyperprolactinemia is usually present to a mild degree, and terminal hair is fine and long, rather than thick and dark. The low chromophore (melanin) content in hair may be another reason for the poor response to hair removal treatments.

8.6. Contraindications for light-based epilation

Absolute contraindications:
- Acute and chronic skin diseases
- Decompensated diabetes mellitus
- Varicose veins at the treatment site
- Severe hypertension and ischemic heart disease

- Acute herpes
- Infectious diseases
- Keloids
- Malignant skin neoplasms

Relative contraindications:
- Pregnancy
- Mental illnesses

The range of specific contraindications for light-based hair removal methods is limited to hypersensitivity to sunlight (photodermatosis).

8.7. Adverse effects associated with light-based epilation

Common side effects of laser hair removal include:
- Persistent pigmentation disorders (hyper- and hypopigmentation)
- Scaling
- Itch
- Erythema
- Edema
- Blisters
- Transient angioectasias
- Pain
- Post-burn scars

Depending on the irradiation power, light can cause various photobiological effects, both thermal (destructive) and biological (stimulating). If the radiation power is insufficient, there is an increased risk of unpredictable effects of irradiation (including increased hair growth) due to triggering a whole range of biological chain processes. On the other hand, excessive radiation power can lead to skin burns. The probability of burns and post-inflammatory hyperpigmentation also increases if patients take drugs with photosensitizing properties.

In some cases, laser hair removal causes a paradoxical increase in hair growth (**paradoxical hypertrichosis**) (Snast I. et al., 2021). Even if hair follicles are mostly destroyed, parts of them can likely persist, regenerate and, in the presence of excess androgens, provide vigorous growth of terminal pigmented hair. This may explain why some women experience paradoxical hypertrichosis after laser epilation.

This condition occurs more often on darker skin and/or after exposure to laser radiation of low energy density. The most common sites for paradoxical hypertrichosis are the chin and neck, with excessive hair growth reported in 6–10% of cases. Paradoxical hypertrichosis is treated with further laser hair removal sessions at high energy densities and with short pulses. It is important to ensure adequate skin cooling to prevent burns.

More information on these topics is available in the *Laser Epilation and Hair Removal Methods in Cosmetic Dermatology & Skincare Practice* book.

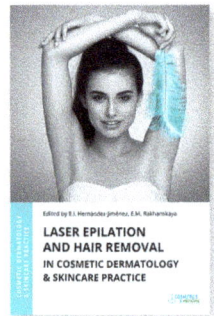

Edited by R.I. Hernandez Jiménez, E.M. Rákhanskaya

LASER EPILATION
AND HAIR REMOVAL
IN COSMETIC DERMATOLOGY
& SKINCARE PRACTICE

Chapter 9
Laser lipolysis

Even though the leading positions among the body shaping methods are still occupied by classical surgical liposuction, laser lipolysis is rapidly gaining market share. Its popularity is increasing because, unlike surgical liposuction, it is minimally traumatic, does not require a long rehabilitation period (some of these procedures are called "lunchtime" treatments, as the patient can do them during lunch break and then return to work) and does not cause serious complications. In addition, device-based methods provide not only lipolysis, but also tightening of the connective tissue framework of the dermis and hypodermis.

Laser lipolysis techniques are either invasive or non-invasive. In the invasive technique, the radiation is delivered directly to the adipose tissue using an optical fiber. In the non-invasive technique, the emitter is located near the skin. In both cases, the aim is to heat the adipose tissue (Lee J.Y. et al., 2021).

9.1. Invasive laser lipolysis

The method is based on inserting a thin cannula under the skin with a fiber-optic light guide which conducts light to the hypodermis and heats fat deposits. The temperature profile in the skin is as follows:

- Hypodermis: 67–68 °C
- Reticular dermis: 44 °C
- Papillary dermis: 42 °C
- Epidermis: up to 41 °C

At these temperatures, the epidermis remains intact. Heating in the dermis leads to the contraction of existing collagen fibers, activation of synthesis of new ones, and restructuring of the dermis. This process manifests as skin thickening and increased skin elasticity in the treatment area.

The most significant damage is observed in the fat, as heating damages the cell membranes of adipocytes, disrupts their barrier function, and causes swelling and lysis. If the liquefied fat emulsion is not removed with a vacuum aspirator, its particles are captured by macrophages, enter the lymphatic vessels, and then metabolize in the liver or are consumed for the body's energy needs.

Interestingly, the overall effectiveness of the invasive laser lipolysis procedure does not depend on whether the destroyed structures are removed immediately during the session by vacuum aspiration or are "processed" by the body — the reduction in the volume of the treated areas will be the same in both cases. Laser lipolysis is currently considered one of the most effective procedures for removing the second chin.

The treatment is performed under local anesthesia and takes about 1–2 hours. After the session, the patient goes home. For the next two weeks, avoiding heavy physical activity is recommended. The effects become noticeable after 2–4 weeks and peak in about three months.

Commercial devices are based on Nd:YAG or Diode lasers (**Table II-9-1**).

Table II-9-1. Devices for invasive laser lipolysis (examples)

TRADE NAME	LASER	WAVELENGTH, nm
SmartLipo (Cynosure, USA)	Nd:YAG	1064
CoolLipo (CoolTouch, USA)	Nd:YAG	1320
ProLipo (Sciton, USA)	Nd:YAG	1064/1319
LipoLite (Syneron, Israel)	Nd:YAG	1064
Lipotherme (Osyris, France)	Diode	980
SlimLipo (Palomar, USA)	Diode	924/975
SmoothLipo (Eleme Medical, USA)	Diode	920
SmartLipo MPX (Cynosure, USA)	Nd:YAG	1064/1320
SmartLipo Triplex (Cynosure, USA)	Nd:YAG	1064/1320/1440

9.2. Non-invasive laser lipolysis

The **non-invasive laser lipolysis** — also known as "cold lipolaser" — relies on **low-level laser radiation (LLLR)** in the red or near-IR spectral range. The most commonly used devices for this purpose are Diode lasers emitting wavelengths from 650 to 900 nm (Avci P. et al., 2013b). At the same time, the power of such radiation is much lower than in conventional laser procedures (in the mW *vs.* W range) and does not lead to significant tissue heating. The emitting tip can be placed directly on or slightly above the skin during the session.

The impact of the LLLR on adipose tissue is not known. According to the initial investigations, micropores are formed in adipocyte membranes, which release lipids from the cell into the extracellular space. Later studies, however, suggested that LLLR activates the complement cascade, triggering adipocyte apoptosis mechanisms. Some authors also believe that, under the action of LLLR, there is a stimulation of mitochondria of fat cells, which causes the activation of ATP formation with further increase in the activity of cyclic adenosine monophosphate (cAMP), protein kinase, and cytoplasmic lipase. The latter breaks down triglycerides into free fatty acids and glycerol. None of these theories have been fully confirmed. However, there are double-blind, placebo-controlled trials showing that LLLR reduces waist circumference, hips, buttocks, and arms. In addition, empirical data show that such an effect reduces the level of cholesterol and triglycerides in the blood serum, which makes this method even more promising. However, authors of all these studies recommend combining non-invasive laser lipolysis procedures using LLLR with interventions that activate microcirculation and lymphatic drainage, as well as physical activity and a healthy diet.

On average, one non-invasive laser lipolysis session takes 40–60 minutes to complete, after which a lymphatic drainage massage (30 to 90 min) is recommended. The procedure is painless and has no recorded side effects. The number of sessions is selected individually: 6–12 procedures spaced by 1–2 days are usually prescribed. Noticeable results can be seen in a week after the course completion.

The 1060-nm Diode laser is also used for non-invasive fat reduction (Schilling L. et al., 2017). This technology is growing in popularity because it yields good clinical results (Fernandez-Nieto D. et al., 2021; Lee J.Y. et al., 2021).

Healthy people with small fat deposits or patients in whom endocrine problems cause obesity are optimal candidates for laser lipolysis. These patients have enough contraindications to preclude using alternative lipolytic techniques.

Chapter 10
Laser-assisted drug delivery

Transdermal delivery of drugs and bioactive compounds involves introducing them into the body through the skin without damaging its barrier structures.

In recent years, ablative fractional photothermolysis with CO_2 lasers has been used in cosmetology to increase the penetration of active compounds into the deep skin layers — the method called **thermoporation (thermoablation)**. This approach allows not only the *stratum corneum* barrier to be "bypassed" but also achieves a synergistic effect of laser radiation and components of cosmetic products, such as rejuvenation procedures, pigment removal, treatment of scars, etc. (Lin C.H. et al., 2014; Wenande E. et al., 2017; Hsiao C.Y. et al., 2019; Bernabe R.M. et al., 2024).

In addition, some studies show that non-ablative fractional laser treatments can increase the skin's permeability to various active substances. It is assumed that such procedures, although not leading to ablation, may create micropores in the *stratum corneum*. Their size is sufficient for the penetration of small molecules but not for large compounds and microorganisms.

Chapter 11
Lasers and hyaluronic fillers

Whether a laser procedure is possible in the area of hyaluronic acid (HA) filler implantation seems a reasonable question. However, more research is needed on this topic.

Hyaluronic fillers are thermostable, but heating can accelerate the rate of their destruction. In the case of laser treatment, the determining factors will be the depth of filler injection and the depth of penetration of the laser beam. If the laser beam "reaches" the filler, heat may destroy it, or its degradation may be accelerated by increased MMP activity. In some cases of unsuccessful filler insertion, laser exposure is intentionally used to remove the implant.

The scientific evidence for combining HA fillers and light-based procedures derives from small and non-randomized studies. Nevertheless, most of these investigations have shown that, on average, the simultaneous use (on the same day) of a laser procedure and fillers represents an effective and safe strategy that improves clinical outcomes and patient satisfaction (Urdiales-Gálvez F. et al., 2019). **Table II-11-1** summarizes some studies on this subject.

According to some sources, if during the session the depth of laser exposure reaches the depth of HA injection (about 2 mm and below), the filler may be damaged by pronounced tissue heating.

However, several authors believe that the depth of action of even the most powerful lasers at 65 °C does not heat the skin in the area of filler implantation to the temperature of its destruction, especially if it is introduced deeply enough to prevent early biodegradation. In addition, as already mentioned, HA is thermostable, since all preparations in the production process are sterilized at temperatures above 120 °C (Bragina I.Y., 2018).

Table II-11-1. Results of clinical and laboratory studies on the combined application of device-based methods and injection of hyaluronic acid-based fillers

STUDY	RESULTS
Ribé A., Ribé N. (2001)	Reduction in the severity of facial wrinkles, as well as improvement of collagen and elastin fiber levels, were noted after HA-based filler injection followed by laser treatment. Laser-induced inflammatory response was observed when using laser radiation of 400–1000 lm (lumen) brightness.
Goldman M.P. et al. (2007)	The study included 26 participants. The nasolabial fold area on one side of the face was subjected to filler injection, and on the other side of the face, the area of filler injection was treated with Diode (1450 nm), Nd:YAG (1320 nm), monopolar RF device, and/or IPL. The reported results indicate that the use of energy-based methods immediately after filler injection did not reduce the overall clinical effect and was safe.
Farkas J.P. et al. (2008)	Hyaluronic filler (three commercial products) was injected into the abdominal skin of pigs. After two weeks, the injection site was treated with one of seven known lasers (ablative or non-ablative). The findings revealed that the injected fillers were not destroyed by non-ablative and slightly ablative (superficial ablative) laser exposure. The more aggressive exposure affected the filler and accelerated its degradation.
Park K.Y. et al. (2011)	The use of IR non-ablative phototherapy in conjunction with HA-based filler injection had no clinical benefits.
Hsu S.H. et al. (2019)	After intradermal injection of HA-based fillers, skin samples obtained during abdominoplasty were treated with fractional laser and micro-needle RF. Laser irradiation did not cause morphologic changes in the filler, while thermal damage was observed along the channels created by micro-needle electrodes.

Even though the most frequently used fractional lasers do not provide such a depth of skin damage, experts recommend adhering to the following recommendations:

1. If a combined procedure (HA filler and phototherapy) is planned on the same day, the process should always start with phototherapy, avoiding skin manipulation after HA-based filler injection. The light radiation must necessarily be characterized by a non-ablative action, minimizing the risk of skin damage and infection.

2. When performing phototherapy as a second step after HA-based filler injection, the use of light sources or lasers with wavelengths exceeding 1000 nm and ms pulse durations should be avoided, especially when preceded by supraperiosteal, mid-dermal, or superficial HA filler injection. In studies on this topic, no problems have been observed when using short-wavelength non-ablative lasers in combination procedures.

3. Phototherapy using radiation with ms, ns, and ps pulse duration, regardless of wavelength, may be performed after injecting any hyaluronic filler.

4. The depth of filler injection is another important aspect to consider when performing a combined procedure on the same day (phototherapy + filler injection). HA-based fillers are injected at different depths, from the supraperiosteal level to the papillary layer of the dermis. That is why it is recommended to perform laser session before HA filler injection.

Chapter 12
Complications associated with laser treatment

The use of any laser method is associated with risk of complications. By complication, we mean a pathologic process or pathologic state that has joined the initial state due to the peculiarities of pathogenesis and/or diagnostic and therapeutic measures (Alster T.S., Li M.K., 2020).

The leading role in preventing complications justifiably belongs to the laser operator that selects patients, chooses the type and parameters of laser radiation, and monitors the recovery and the patient's degree of compliance. **The operator must timely and adequately manage the pathological process in case of its occurrence, minimizing the likely adverse consequences.**

Risks of complications depend on:
- Selection of device and parameters of laser treatment
- Operator's sequence of action
- Patient characteristics

The analysis of complications due to laser treatments facilitates the optimization of therapy protocols. However, as statistical data and information on the complications associated with laser treatments are poorly presented, it is customary to consider adverse reactions mainly based on their clinical manifestations (Kalashnikova N.G. et al., 2021).

Classification based on etiologic factors includes the following groups of complications:
1. Mistakes in selecting patients for laser treatment
2. Wrong choice of laser equipment
3. Incorrect laser radiation parameters
4. Violation of procedural protocol
5. Inadequate post-procedure care
6. Individual patient's reaction to laser radiation

12.1. Mistakes in selecting patients for laser treatment

1. **No prior examination to exclude malignant and precancerous lesions, which are an absolute contraindication for laser treatment due to the possible risk of their progression.**

   Malignant and precancerous lesions with cutaneous localization may be missed due to errors in differential diagnosis and neglect of additional examination methods, particularly dermatoscopy.

   Malignant and precancerous neoplasms with internal localization and accompanying skin symptoms may not be diagnosed due to the physician's inadequate assessment of the patient's general somatic status.

   For example, lanuginous hypertrichosis usually begins with increased hair growth in the face and is characterized by further spread of the process to other parts of the body, prompting the patient to seek laser hair removal. Lack of oncologic vigilance, inattention to the history, and failure to conduct comprehensive assessment of the patient's somatic status lead to untimely diagnosis, lack of complete therapy and, as a consequence, adverse effect on the patient's health.

2. **The pathogenetic features of the skin process exposed to laser treatment are not taken into account.**

   Dermatological problems may be a manifestation of systemic pathology (congenital syndromes, autoimmune and endocrine diseases, etc.). Laser treatment is ineffective in these cases, but may stimulate the activity of the pathological process. At present, the safety of laser methods in these conditions is under research.

   Local skin pathology with a progressive course and high sensitivity to external factors can result in rapid neoplasm growth triggered by laser exposure.

3. **Incorrect choice of laser device.**

   Although laser-based methods are widely used in practice as monotherapy, they are not considered the first line of recommended therapy in cases of significant severity and torpid course of the skin process, as they may yield unsatisfactory results and cause disease progression.

4. **Underestimating the importance or ignoring the risk factors for developing predictable adverse reactions often provokes the subsequent addition of another pathologic process to the patient's original condition.**

Risk factors for severe adverse conditions:
- Concomitant somatic pathology (hypertensive crisis, bronchospasm, epilepsy, etc.)
- "Local" problems (systemic allergic reaction when QS lasers fragment tattoo pigment, which causes the formation of allergic granuloma)

Risk factors for the development of local complications in the area of exposure:
- Dark skin phototype or tanned skin
- Tendency toward pathologic scarring
- Recurrent infections (viral, bacterial, fungal)
- Bad habits that reduce the regeneration rate
- Previously administered exogenous drugs and substances
- Other factors that sometimes remain unidentified

Preventive measures at the stage of patient selection for laser therapy:
1. Differential diagnosis with a careful collection of anamnesis, comprehensive assessment of somatic status, and oncologic vigilance
2. Identification and exclusion of patients with contraindications for laser treatment methods and risk factors for complications
3. Making a prospective prognosis of the risks and effectiveness of laser treatment considering nosology, its pathogenesis, clinical manifestations, laboratory examination data, and current treatment recommendations
4. Informed choice of the optimal treatment strategy for each patient, namely:
   - Laser application as a part of complex therapy (taking into account the specifics of interaction between different methods)
   - Laser treatment as monotherapy
   - Rejection of laser therapy

12.2. Improper selection of equipment

1. Using uncertified devices the safety of which has not been confirmed and results cannot be predicted.
2. Unjustified use of non-selective methods involving the removal of the target and surrounding tissues contributes to an increased risk of complications.
3. Violation of the principle of selective photothermolysis: the use of "pseudoselective" methods has a pronounced effect not only on the target but also on the surrounding tissues, causing their overheating and subsequent formation of de-, hypo-, and hyperpigmentation, burns, and scars.

Selection of a suboptimal wavelength (non-observance of optical selectivity): laser radiation is more effectively absorbed by competitive chromophores outside the target. For example, the effect of ALEX radiation not only on hair melanin but also on skin melanin during hair removal in patients with high skin phototype often results in pigmentation disorders. Similarly, owing to its insufficient penetrating ability, laser radiation is absorbed mainly in the upper layers of the skin by hemoglobin in the small capillaries and melanin, causing superficial burns without yielding the desired therapeutic effect on the target dilated vessels.

Inadequate choice of laser radiation generation mode (failure to observe thermal selectivity) leads to laser pulse duration that exceeds the thermal relaxation time of the target and provides conditions for complication development.

Preventive measures at the stage of selecting laser treatment equipment:
1. Use of certified devices for registered indications.
2. Selective therapies should be favored in the absence of contraindications.
3. Laser radiation should be chosen to ensure **optical selectivity** (its absorption efficiency by target chromophores should be higher than that of other endogenous chromophores in

the surrounding tissues) and penetration to the depth of the target object.
4. Application of devices with the mode of radiation generation corresponding to the peculiarities of the target, to comply with the conditions of **thermal selectivity** (pulse duration should be shorter than the TRT of the target) and to prevent excessive heat outflow into the adjacent tissues.

12.3. Incorrect laser parameters

It should be noted that the following causes of complications are the **most common**:
1. Technical issues with the device (disconnection, damage or contamination of lenses, shutter breakage, cooling system dysfunction, etc.) cause treatment programs to fail and outgoing radiation parameters to deviate from the declared ones. As a result, physical and biological processes occurring in the treatment zone will differ from the expected ones and will have other clinical effects.
2. Incorrect choice of physical parameters of laser radiation (energy density, duration of exposure, spot size), not corresponding to the features of the target object, leads to traumatization of the surrounding tissues.

Preventive measures at the stage of selection of physical parameters of laser radiation for the treatment session:
1. The operator has special knowledge of the basics of laser physics, as well as the ability to analyze the relationship between changes in the physical parameters of laser radiation and biophysical processes occurring in tissues under its influence.
2. Diagnostics of equipment serviceability before each work shift, control of optics cleanliness and operating rules, regular timely maintenance, categorical refusal to work with faulty equipment.
3. Step-by-step selection of energy parameters, focusing not on the recommended digital values, but on visual tissue changes

occurring in the treatment zone and their compliance with the changes required from the clinical point of view.

4. Immediate procedure termination in case of undesirable phenomena followed by a detailed analysis of causes, with continuation of work only after their elimination.

12.4. Violation of procedure protocol

1. Non-compliance with safety rules during laser therapy is associated with the following risk factors for complications:
   - High voltage: the possibility of wiring fire and extreme situations.
   - High energy in the area of exposure: contact with flammable objects (hair, clothing, etc.) may also cause fire and burns.
   - Direct and reflected laser radiation can cause ocular complications in the absence of eye protection: damage to the anterior media with 180–380 nm and >1400 nm radiation; damage to the posterior media of the eye when 380–1400 nm wavelengths are used.
   - Tissue vapor products irritate the mucous membranes of the upper respiratory tract and contribute to viral infection.
   - If there is a wound in the laser treatment area, it may become infected after the procedure.

2. The treatment area is not adequately prepared. The presence of foreign impurities on the skin surface (most often cosmetic particles that have unknown spectral properties and may act as a competing chromophore) leads to the loss of selectivity and unpredictable results.

3. Errors in the application of skin surface treatment technique:
   - **Incorrect positioning of the manipulator** causes laser radiation to be transmitted from the slice of the light guide instead of its end surface. As a result, tissues located near the area of exposure are damaged.

- **Non-compliance with the scanning mode of treatment with repeated exposure of the same body area to the beam** leads to complications such as scar formation.
- **Absence of test treatment** with the chosen exposure settings may lead to aesthetically unacceptable results on a large area, such as when removing a permanent tattoo.

Preventive measures during a laser session:
1. Strict observance of safety protocols and use of protective equipment (goggles, gloves, masks, ventilation, aseptic and antiseptic rules).
2. Keeping the treatment area free of any cosmetics for 12 hours (due to the penetration of particles into the skin pores), thorough cleansing of the treatment area.
3. Training of specialists and strict adherence to the procedure protocol (location of the manipulator, treatment mode and number of passes, application of the light spot, etc.).
4. Conducting a test procedure on a small area in case of a doubtful result of exposure in order to be able to further evaluate the response and make an informed decision on further strategies.

12.5. Inadequate post-procedure care

1. Insufficient or unconvincing information about the importance of following standard recommendations during rehabilitation reduces patient compliance, leads to violations of the regimen in the post-procedure period and, consequently, increases the risk of complications. For example, depending on the type of laser treatment, patient may be advised to avoid sunbathing, water exposure, heat-based procedures, traumatization, friction, wearing close-fitting clothing, etc. Neglecting the recommendations, in particular the advice to avoid insolation, causes increased pigmentation.
2. The absence of preventive antiviral and antibacterial therapy when indicated (treatment of areas "at risk" of herpetic infection, frequently recurring herpes, non-stable acne remission, etc.) may result in the generalization of local infection.

Preventive measures for the management in the post-procedure period:

Fully informing the patient (orally and in writing, with hand-delivered instructions) on the following issues:

1. Justification of care recommendations and the likelihood of negative consequences if they are violated.
2. A description of the clinical picture of the normal post-procedure period and abnormalities for which immediate medical attention should be sought.
3. Prescribing gentle, proven treatments after aggressive procedures.
4. Preventive therapy for infection (if warranted).

12.6. Individual reactions to laser radiation

The following list is the least predictable group of complications, which usually cannot be prevented.

1. **Response to laser radiation exposure**

   Local:
   - Urticarial follicular reaction after epilation
   - Paradoxical hypertrichosis
   - Leukotrichia
   - Photodermatitis

   Systemic:
   - Lupus erythematosus
   - Dermatomyositis

2. **Reaction to the combination of laser radiation with other factors.** There are known cases when, on the second day of the Er:YAG + SMA facial treatment, after double application of aqueous chlorhexidine solution, a pronounced facial edema developed, and against the background of anticoagulant treatment, petechial rash appeared in the treatment area.

Summarizing the analysis, the following should be noted:

- The complications that can occur after laser treatment are very diverse and have a wide range of causes.
- Such complications arise even in the practice of experienced physicians, but their probability depends on the professional expertise and diligence of the specialist.
- The doctor's understanding of the principles of physical and biological interaction of laser radiation with tissues significantly reduces the risk of adverse reactions.
- Analysis of previous complications allows the development and application of preventive measures.
- The preventive approach should be comprehensive and must be implemented at every stage of treatment.

Equipment innovations, improvements in the existing technologies, continuous improvement of professional knowledge of cosmetologists, understanding and prevention of potential complications, and their early recognition and mitigation significantly contribute to the greater safety of laser methods.

Part III

Organizational matters

Chapter 1
Laser safety

1.1. Laser hazard classes

Working with lasers requires special attention in terms of safety. Accordingly, rules and regulations about lasers are in force worldwide.

These rules determine the safety measures required for people who might be exposed to lasers and classify lasers based on their potential risks.

There are two classification systems: the "old system" that was in use prior to 2002 and the "revised system" introduced in 2002, reflecting increased knowledge about lasers. The revised system is part of the IEC 60825 standard and was also incorporated into the U.S.-oriented ANSI Laser Safety Standard (ANSI Z136.1) in 2007.

The laser classification is determined based on accessible emission limits (AELs). These limits are defined for each laser class and typically specify the maximum power (in watts, W) or energy (in joules, J) the laser can emit within a specified wavelength range and exposure time. This measurement is taken through a defined aperture stop at a specified distance.

For infrared wavelengths beyond 4 µm, the AEL is specified as a maximum power density (in watts per square meter, W/m^2). Lasers are classified according to their wavelength and power, ranging from Class 1 (no hazard during normal use) to Class 4 (severe hazard for eyes and skin).

Manufacturers are responsible for correctly classifying lasers, providing appropriate warning labels, and following safety measures outlined by regulations. Safety measures for powerful lasers include key-controlled operation, warning lights for laser emission, a beam stop or attenuator, and an electrical contact for emergency stops or interlocks.

These precautions are crucial to ensure the safe handling and operation of lasers, particularly in industrial, medical, and scientific settings where higher-powered lasers are commonly used.

IEC 60825-1 is an international standard that outlines the characteristics and requirements for the laser classification system (**Table III-1-1**). The main features are presented below:

1. Accessible Emission Limit (AEL): Specifies the maximum power or energy emitted in a defined wavelength range, exposure time, and through a specified aperture at a certain distance.
2. Classification system:
   - Class 1: No hazard during normal use.
   - Class 1M, 2M, 3R, 3B, 4: Hazardous, with increasing severity from 1M to 4.
3. Warning labels:
   - Class 1: Typically, no specific warning label is required.
   - Class 1M, 2M, 3R, 3B, 4: Triangular warning label is mandatory.
4. Additional labels:
   - Other labels are required in specific cases, indicating laser emission, laser apertures, skin hazards, and invisible wavelengths.

Table III-1-1. IEC 60825-1 classification of laser devices

CLASS	DESCRIPTION
1	**CLASS 1 LASER PRODUCT** A Class 1 laser is considered safe for all normal use conditions. This means that the Maximum Permissible Exposure (MPE) limit is not exceeded when viewing the laser with the naked eye or using typical magnifying optics like a telescope or microscope. To ensure compliance, the standard specifies the aperture and distance corresponding to the naked eye, a standard telescope viewing a collimated beam, and a typical microscope viewing a divergent beam. **Medical applications:** • Diagnostics • Laser therapy

Continued on p. 173

CLASS	DESCRIPTION
1M	

LASER RADIATION
DO NOT VIEW DIRECTLY WITH OPTICAL INSTRUMENTS
CLASS 1M LASER PRODUCT

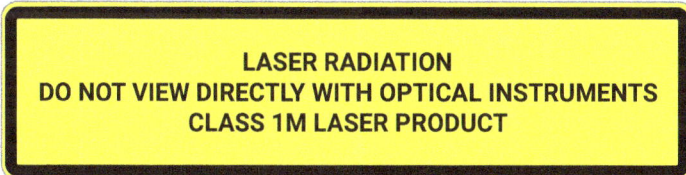

A Class 1M laser is generally safe for all regular usage scenarios, except when the beam is passed through magnifying optics like microscopes and telescopes. Class 1M lasers typically produce large-diameter or divergent beams. The MPE for a Class 1M laser is usually not exceeded unless the beam is focused or imaged using optics to make it narrower. If the beam is refocused, this could increase the hazard associated with Class 1M lasers, potentially leading to a change in the product class. A laser is classified as Class 1M if the power passing through the pupil of the naked eye is below the Accessible Emission Limit (AEL) for Class 1. Still, the power collected into the eye by typical magnifying optics (as defined in the standard) is higher than the AEL for Class 1 and lower than the AEL for Class 3B. This classification system helps ensure appropriate safety considerations, especially when dealing with lasers that may pose risks when viewed through magnifying devices.

Medical applications:

- Diagnostics
- Laser therapy

2

LASER RADIATION
DO NOT STARE INTO BEAM
CLASS 2 LASER PRODUCT

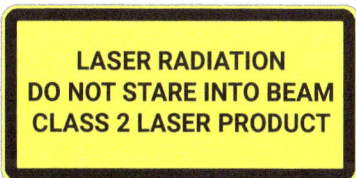

A Class 2 laser is considered safe because of the natural blink reflex, an automatic response of the body to bright lights, which limits exposure to no more than 0.25 seconds. This classification specifically applies to visible-light lasers with a wavelength ranging from 400 to 700 nanometers. Class 2 lasers are restricted to a maximum continuous power of 1 milliwatt (mW), or more if the emission time is less than 0.25 seconds or if the light is not spatially coherent. Intentionally suppressing the blink reflex could lead to eye injury.

Medical applications:

- Laser therapy

Continued on p. 174

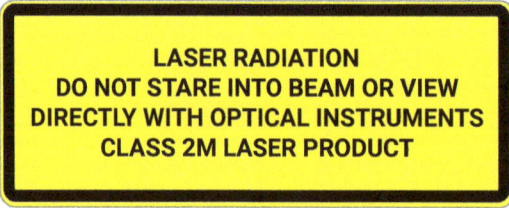

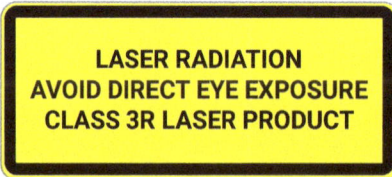

CLASS	DESCRIPTION
2M	**LASER RADIATION** **DO NOT STARE INTO BEAM OR VIEW** **DIRECTLY WITH OPTICAL INSTRUMENTS** **CLASS 2M LASER PRODUCT** A Class 2M laser is considered safe due to the blink reflex if not viewed through optical instruments. Similar to Class 1M, this safety classification applies to laser beams with a large diameter or large divergence. The safety assurance comes from the fact that, if directly viewed, the amount of light passing through the pupil cannot exceed the limits specified for Class 2 lasers. It is crucial to avoid using optical instruments, as they can focus or concentrate the laser beam, potentially increasing the risk of eye injury. As long as these lasers are used in accordance with safety guidelines, they pose minimal risk to the eyes. **Medical applications:** • Laser therapy
3R	**LASER RADIATION** **AVOID DIRECT EYE EXPOSURE** **CLASS 3R LASER PRODUCT** A Class 3R laser is considered safe when handled carefully, with restrictions on direct beam viewing. Although the MPE for a Class 3R laser can be exceeded, the risk of injury is low. Specifically, visible continuous lasers within Class 3R are limited to 5 milliwatts (mW). Different limits apply for lasers of other wavelengths and for pulsed lasers. Users need to exercise caution and follow safety guidelines when working with Class 3R lasers. While they pose a lower risk than higher-class lasers, precautions should still be taken to minimize the potential for accidental exposure and ensure safe usage. **Medical applications:** • Laser therapy • PDT

Continued on p. 175

CLASS	DESCRIPTION
3B	**LASER RADIATION** **AVOID EXPOSURE TO BEAM** **CLASS 3B LASER PRODUCT** A Class 3B laser is considered hazardous if the eye is directly exposed to its beam, but reflections from matte surfaces, like paper, are generally not harmful. The AEL for continuous lasers in the wavelength range from 315 nm to far infrared is 0.5 W. For pulsed lasers operating between 400 and 700 nm, the limit is 30 millijoules (mJ). Different limits apply to lasers of other wavelengths and to ultrashort-pulsed lasers. Protective eyewear is typically required in situations where there is a possibility of direct viewing of a Class 3B laser beam. Class 3B lasers are also required to have a key switch and a safety interlock for additional safety measures. **Medical applications:** • Laser therapy • PDT
4	**LASER RADIATION** **AVOID EYE OR SKIN EXPOSURE TO** **DIRECT OR SCATTERED RADIATION** **CLASS 4 LASER PRODUCT** Class 4 lasers represent the highest and most dangerous category, encompassing all lasers that exceed the AEL of Class 3B. A Class 4 laser has the potential to cause severe and permanent damage to the skin and eyes through direct, diffuse, or indirect viewing of the beam. In addition, these lasers can ignite combustible materials, presenting a significant fire risk. Hazards may also arise from indirect or non-specular reflections of the beam, even from apparently matte surfaces. This emphasizes the critical importance of carefully controlling the beam path. For safety reasons, Class 4 lasers must be equipped with a key switch and a safety interlock. Medical lasers may have divergent emissions, requiring awareness of the nominal ocular hazard distance (NOHD) and nominal ocular hazard area (NOHA) to prevent accidental exposure. Due to the severe risks associated with Class 4 lasers, strict safety measures and protocols must be followed during their operation and handling. **Medical applications:** • PDT • Laser surgery

1.2. Health risks

An important feature of working with lasers is seasonality. The most active procedures are performed in the fall, winter, and spring. This time coincides with the period when the central heating is on and the temperature in the working area of medical offices rises. In addition, the use of heating devices and air conditioners reduces the oxygen concentration in the room, which adversely affects the well-being of medical personnel, resulting in:

- Decreased performance and drowsiness
- Quick onset of fatigue
- Decreased concentration
- Headaches and blood pressure changes
- Dryness of mucous membranes of the nasopharynx, which leads to decreased resistance to viral infections and exacerbation of bacterial infections
- Dryness of the mucous membranes of the eye, which may cause conjunctivitis and compromise vision

All this significantly affects the state of health, reducing the body's immunity. Laser radiation poses the greatest threat to the retina and anterior media of the eye (**Table III-1-2**), as well as to the exposed skin of the neck, thyroid gland, and mammary glands.

Table III-1-2. Types of damage to the eyes caused by laser radiation depending on wavelength

RANGE	WAVELENGTH (nm)	TYPE OF DAMAGE
UVC	100–280	• Keratoconjunctivitis • Erythema of the eyelid skin
UVB	280–315	• Keratoconjunctivitis • Erythema of the eyelid skin • Cataract
UVA	315–400	• Keratoconjunctivitis • Cataract • Damage to the retina

Continued on p. 177

RANGE	WAVELENGTH (nm)	TYPE OF DAMAGE
Visible light	400–780	• Photochemical damage to the retina by blue light • Thermal burns of the retina and the ocular vasculature proper • Thermal burns to the iris of the eye
IR-A	780–1400	• Thermal burns of the retina and the ocular vasculature proper • Cataract
IR-B	1400–3000	• Burning of the eyelid skin
IR-C	3000–10,000	• Corneal burns • Conjunctival burns

Harmful and hazardous factors of the working environment when operating lasers are summarized in **Table III-1-3**.

Table III-1-3. Harmful and hazardous factors of the working environment when operating lasers

UNFAVOR-ABLE FACTORS	SOURCES (CAUSE) OF OCCURRENCE	LASER HAZARD CLASS			
		1	2	3	4
Direct laser light	Laser (active body) — particularly relevant for alignment work	–	+	+	+
Diffusely and mirror scattered laser radiation	Laser beam interaction: • with various elements along the beam path (smooth surface of the target, glass, finishing tiles, oil paint covering walls and partitions) • with airborne particles	–	–	+	+
Pulsed light flashes	• Radiation from pulsed pump lamps without shields • Plasma plume radiation	–	–	– (+)	+
UV radiation	• Radiation from pulsed pump lamps • Quartz discharge tubes and cuvettes	–	–	– (+)	+

Continued on p. 178

UNFAVOR-ABLE FACTORS	SOURCES (CAUSE) OF OCCURRENCE	LASER HAZARD CLASS			
		1	2	3	4
Ozone, nitrogen oxides and other chemical factors, including aerosols	• Air ionization at discharge of pulse pump lamps • Active medium (e.g., phosphorus oxychloride) in liquid lasers • Coolant (in case of careless handling when changing coolant) • Destruction products of laser beam-treated materials	–	–	– (+)	+
Noise, vibration	• Operation of auxiliary elements of the laser installation (cooling system, local exhaust ventilation systems, etc.) • Sound pulses from the laser beam hitting the target can reach up to 100–120 dB at a frequency of 125–400 Hz (up to several hundred pulses per shift)	–	–	– (+)	+
Soft X-rays and neutron radiation	• Laser operating voltage over 10 kV, interaction of high-power laser radiation with the target	–	–	– (+)	+
Radiofrequency (RF) electromagnetic fields	• High-frequency and ultra-high-frequency laser pumping	–	–	–	– (+)
Elevated surface temperatures	• Target material	–	–	– (+)	+

1.3. How to ensure safe work with lasers in clinical practice

Safety when working with lasers is ensured through collective and personal protective equipment (PPE), which must meet the accepted standards and safety measures for the device.

The heads of medical institutions are responsible for the fulfillment of all requirements. They are responsible for the creation and approval of precise instructions to be followed when performing laser procedures.

These instructions should include the specific names of laser devices and the names of the units (rooms) in which these devices are located. An example of such a document is given below.

INSTRUCTION
on the operation and safety rules when working with laser devices

General provisions

1. Depending on the aser hazard class, the following adverse factors may affect personnel:
   - Laser light is direct, mirror-like
   - Light emission
   - Infrared radiation
   - Gases and aerosols
   - High- and ultra-high-frequency electromagnetic fields
   - Ionizing radiation at operating voltages above 10 kV
2. Only persons not younger than 18 years old with completed higher and secondary vocational education, who have a certificate of special training course completion, who have studied technical documentation, instructions on the rules of operation, labor protection and safety during the operation of the installation, and instructions on first aid in case of accidents, who have been instructed directly at the workplace, are allowed to work on laser devices.
3. Fire safety regulations must be observed in rooms where work on laser machines is carried out.
4. The installation and its design must ensure that the operating personnel cannot come in direct contact with the power source when it is switched on. The installation must have alarms and interlocks to ensure the safety of the operating personnel.
5. Every work-related accident must be reported immediately by the victim or an eyewitness of the accident to the supervisor,

who must organize first aid to the victim, his/her transportation to a medical institution, and inform the head of the institution, the occupational safety engineer or a person performing his/her functions, and the trade union committee about the incident. It is necessary to preserve for investigation the situation at the workplace and the state of the equipment as it was at the time of the incident, if doing so does not threaten the life and health of the surrounding workers and will not lead to an accident.

Safety measures

1. The installation uses a laser (*specify type*); in terms of hazard, the generated radiation belongs to the (*specify hazard class*) hazard class.
2. The sources of danger are:
   - 220 V AC voltage in the power supply circuits of the laser power supply control unit
   - Voltage over 1 kV in the high-voltage connector
   - Laser radiation (direct, mirror-reflected)
3. The doors of the room should have a "Do Not Enter" sign and a laser hazard sign that reads "Caution, Laser Radiation."
4. Instruments and objects with mirrored surfaces must not be used in the room where the unit is located. The tools used in work must have a matte surface.
5. Personnel working with laser devices must use the necessary personal protective equipment (PPE) in accordance with the requirements determined by the laser hazard class.
6. In the room with laser devices where ozone, nitrogen oxides or other harmful gases, vapors and aerosols may be formed, forced supply and exhaust ventilation shall be provided to reduce their content in the air to the concentration allowed by sanitary norms.
7. Illumination (natural and artificial) should correspond to the optimal values defined in the relevant instructions.
8. The personnel shall immediately report all laser malfunctions, noncompliance of PPE with the requirements, and other deviations from the normal operating mode to the administration and record them in the operating log.

Forbidden activities

1. When working with laser light it is mandatory not to:
   - Look toward the primary and mirror-reflected ray
   - Leave the space in which manipulation is performed uncontrolled
   - Work without protective goggles in the radiation area
   - Carry out repair and adjustment work with the unit connected to the mains
2. When operating the device it is forbidden to:
   - Replace mains fuses, connect and disconnect cables while the unit is plugged in
   - Observe direct or specular reflection of laser radiation
   - Work on a known defective machine
   - Leave the unit unattended when it is switched on
   - Use homemade and non-standard fuses
   - Disconnect the high-voltage connector earlier than 2 min after disconnecting the laser power supply from the mains
   - Turn on the laser with the power supply transmitter connector undocked
3. Use cord with damaged insulation
4. Drop the cord to avoid breaking the plug
5. Plug the system into the mains if the mains socket does not meet the requirements of the protection class of the system
6. Operate the unit in rooms with a relative humidity exceeding 80%
7. Install fuses that do not correspond to the rated value

The instruction should also specify the person responsible for the safe operation of laser equipment with reference to the relevant internal regulations issued by the administration of the medical institution.

1.4. General precautions for working with lasers

To reduce the risk of occupational hazards and to maintain health while working with a laser apparatus, the operator must take appropriate precautions. Despite the variety of procedures performed with laser systems, it is possible to formulate common approaches that contribute to the organization of a safe work process, as exemplified below.

1. Procedures should only be carried out in a specially equipped room with adequate:
    - Lighting (daylight lamps, magnifying lamps)
    - Ventilation
2. While using lasers, it is necessary to:
    - Ventilate the room after each procedure (timely ventilation of the room will improve air exchange, reduce the temperature and humidity in the working area to normal, and reduce the concentration of viruses and bacteria in the air)
    - Use personal protective equipment (PPE) — goggles, masks, gloves, armbands, protective clothing against heat radiation, etc.
    - Prevent the laser housing from overheating
    - Not direct the laser beam sideways
    - Remove all fibrous materials and flammable surfaces (cotton disks, gauze, paper napkins, spatulas, etc.) from the beam's path
    - Take regular breaks from work
    - Wet-clean the office at least twice a day

Each laser method has its own characteristics which will determine additional professional protection measures that must be adopted.

1.5. Additional precautions for laser procedures

1.5.1. Fractional laser thermolysis, "laser resurfacing"

Specialists performing this procedure face a complex set of harmful factors:
- Vapors containing oxides and "bio-dust"
- Possibility of contact with skin fragments, blood, mucus, saliva

- Smoke from the destruction of skin neoplasms and carbonization products

Recommendations
- Remove ablation products from the patient's skin during the procedure
- Use smoke evacuators
- Use protective clothing to prevent overheating, in addition to conventional PPE

1.5.2. Laser coagulation of vessels

This procedure raises the temperature in the work area above the permissible values.

Recommendations
- Use units with built-in cooling system
- Control the air humidity
- Ensure that heat is removed from the patient's skin (cold packs)

1.5.3. Carbon peel

The following hazards are associated with this procedure:
- Carbon dust, smoke
- Industrial noise
- Vibration
- Increased content of nitrogen compounds in the air

Recommendations
- Use additional PPE — protective aprons with a surface suitable for wet processing
- Provide protection for eyes, nasopharynx and mucous membranes, respiratory tract, exposed skin
- Only perform procedures in rooms with supply and exhaust ventilation
- Carefully remove carbon residue from the skin surface

1.5.4. Photodynamic therapy

When performing this procedure, professionals are exposed to the following harmful factors:
- Increased eye strain
- ROS, ozone, nitrogenous compounds
- Forced posture

Recommendations
- Use additional PPE — overalls that cover exposed areas of the chest and neck (thyroid area)
- Air the place out more often

1.5.5. Laser removal of tattoos and permanent makeup

Harmful factors:
- Noise (photoacoustic effect)
- Vibration
- Smoke
- Release of dye degradation products
- Temperature increase in the working area

Recommendations
- Use smoke evacuators
- Use additional PPE — overalls that cover exposed skin

It should be noted that non-compliance with these sanitary rules and regulations, as well as practical guidelines, can be harmful to health or lead to disability.

1.6. Basics of first aid

Operators of laser installations should have "Instructions for first aid in case of eye and skin damage by laser radiation" in their work area. An example of such instructions is given below.

INSTRUCTION
on the first aid for eye injury and skin with laser radiation

If the rules of laser operation are not followed, the radiation may cause eye damage. The severity and nature of the damage depend on the radiation wavelength, its energy, duration of exposure, and other conditions.

Exposure to ultraviolet (180 to 315 nm) or infrared (above 1400 nm) laser radiation may cause corneal damage. Exposure to visible (in the 380–780 nm range) or near-IR (780–1400 nm) laser radiation may cause damage to the retina.

When the cornea is damaged, there is eye pain, eyelid spasm, lacrimation, hyperemia of the mucous membranes of the eyelids and eyeball, their edema, edema of the corneal epithelium, and erosions. Severe corneal damage is accompanied by clouding of the anterior chamber fluid.

In mild retinal damage, a small area of opaque retina is observed on the eye fundus. In severe cases, there is an area of retinal necrosis, retinal tissue rupture, and the retina may be ejected into the vitreous body. These injuries are accompanied by hemorrhage into the retina, pre- or subretinal spaces , or vitreous body.

First aid for corneal injury consists of applying a sterile dressing to the injured eye and referring the victim to an eye hospital.

In retinal damage, timely first aid is aimed at creating favorable conditions for the formation of chorioretinal scar by reducing secondary phenomena accompanying the damage, and by weakening tissue edema.

First aid in retinal damage:
- Intravenous injection of 40% glucose solution (20 ml) with the addition of 0.1% suprastin solution (1 ml) or
- Intravenous injection of 10% sodium chloride solution (10 ml), intravenous dimedrol (0.1 g)

After receiving first aid, the victim is referred to an eye hospital.

When working with laser radiation, open areas of the body — the skin — are also exposed to danger. It is important to note that the energy of powerful laser radiation can affect the skin even if covered by some textile materials. In addition, there is a possibility of clothing ignition in contact with the laser beam. The severity of damage to the skin and in some cases the whole organism depends on the energy of radiation, duration of exposure, area of damage, its localization, and presence of secondary sources of exposure (burning, smoldering). Contact with laser radiation produces a sensation of heat or pain. The pain intensity depends on the skin lesion area. Skin damage by laser radiation energy in the UV spectral range (non-thermal energy levels) can occur without any sensations.

The nature of skin lesions when exposed to laser radiation is similar to thermal burns. Depending on the level of the applied energy, erythema, pale area (coagulation necrosis), dry and wet vesicles (detachment of horny scales and the entire epidermis), charring of the upper skin layers, and funnel-shaped depressions (in case of a focused beam) may appear on the skin surface.

Laser skin burns, like thermal burns, can be categorized by the depth of injury into the following four grades:

Grade 1: erythema of the skin

Grade 2: the appearance of blisters

Grade 3a: necrosis of the superficial skin layers

Grade 3b: necrosis of the entire skin thickness

Grade 4: tissue necrosis at varying depths beyond the skin

The nature of therapeutic measures in laser skin burns is determined not only by the depth, but also by the extent of skin damage. First aid should be aimed at preventing contamination and traumatization of the burned surfaces.

First aid measures in skin burns caused by laser include:

1. In the event of a clothing fire, quickly extinguish the flames and remove smoldering textile material
2. Immediately cool the skin lesion area (water, ice) for a few minutes, which will reduce the depth of the burn by one degree
3. Put on a dry sterile dressing
4. In case of deep and extensive skin burns, anesthetics should be administered
5. Refer the victim to a surgeon at the nearest medical facility

1.7. Home lasers

In recent years, many portable devices for home use called "laser" have appeared on the market. Portable devices cannot achieve high energy parameters due to the low power of diode emitters. This leads to an increase in the number of treatments and exposure time, affecting the dose/effect ratio. Uncontrolled use of "home lasers" may thus cause health problems.

Clinical manifestations of chronic exposure to low-intensity electromagnetic waves are divided into two groups.

1. **Early signs:**
   - Rapid fatigue
   - Irritability
   - Sleep disturbance
   - Headaches

2. **Late signs:**
   - Pain in the heart area, sometimes similar to angina pectoris
   - Decreased appetite
   - Vegetovascular disorders with a vascular component (hypotension), pulse lability, tendency to arterial hypertension and angiospastic reactions, narrowing of retinal arteries
   - Nightmarish dreams, intrusive thoughts
   - Trophic and endocrine disorders (decreased body weight, hair loss, brittle nails, thyroid hyperfunction, impotence, increased histamine and blood sugar levels, moderate dysproteinemia, decreased blood cholinesterase levels, impaired catecholamine release)

The use of lasers has become an integral part of modern skincare, cosmetic dermatology, and aesthetic medicine, but in an effort to increase the effectiveness of laser therapy, one should not forget about the observance of safety rules when working with laser installations. These rules should be followed by managers of medical institutions as well as by all personnel.

Chapter 2
Selecting a laser for the practice

Lasers are high-tech, expensive devices that allow solving a variety of dermatological and aesthetic problems. However, in some cases, the purchased equipment may be unreasonably idle or its capabilities are not fully utilized, which leads to loss of investment benefits. Accordingly, informed choice of laser devices is vital for medical business owners and managers. This choice should not only be based on the distributors' statements, but should also take into account many other aspects, including the demand and profitability of procedures, doctors' qualifications and willingness to work with lasers, actual technical characteristics of the devices, specifics of the location and specialization of the institution, etc.

This section has been prepared on the basis of more than 25 years of experience with laser equipment. We present some practical points that may help practitioners planning to invest in a laser in selecting the most suitable device and optimizing its performance.

2.1. Applications of lasers in dermatology and aesthetic medicine

- Skin rejuvenation, wrinkle removal
- Scar and striae revision
- Hair removal
- Vascular lesion therapy
- Pigment lesion therapy
- Tattoo removal
- Skin neoplasm removal
- Acne treatment

- Treatment of certain dermatologic pathologies (e.g., vitiligo, psoriasis)
- Laser-assisted lipolysis or liposuction
- Gynecology (treatment and prevention of vaginal relaxation syndrome, urinary incontinence, genital prolapse, aesthetics of labia and skin)
- Minimally invasive skin tightening
- Phlebology (endovenous laser photocoagulation)
- Onychomycosis therapy

There are certain areas in which the use of lasers is most optimal, such as laser hair removal, which is considered an accepted global standard for hair removal and ranks first in the rating of demand for device-based interventions and third among all non-invasive cosmetic procedures, second only to botulinum toxin and hyaluronic acid injections. The absence of such a highly effective procedure in a cosmetology clinic can cause client bewilderment and may negatively affect the institution's reputation. Therefore, the justification of investment in a laser hair removal device does not raise any particular questions.

But if we are talking, for example, about wrinkle removal or skin rejuvenation in general, then in case of a limited budget, the question arises whether this particular medical center needs the appropriate laser or not, if the list of services already includes other methods of correcting age-related changes. It should be understood that there are different targets for the correction of age-related changes in the skin and subcutaneous structures. On the one hand, the use of laser does not eliminate the need for the correction of dynamic wrinkles with botulinum toxin, volume plastics, etc. On the other hand, the use of injectable methods will not result in the skin condition achieved by laser rejuvenation, so a full correction of age-related changes should include laser exposure. In the case of other indications, in some situations the use of lasers is "highly specific," i.e., the efficiency and cost-effectiveness of procedures justifies the high cost of lasers, and in other cases the decision should be made depending on the specific conditions (**Table III-2-1**).

Table III-2-1. Some applications of lasers in dermatology and aesthetic medicine

SCOPE OF APPLICATION		DEGREE OF SPECIFICITY OF THE LASER TREATMENT	ALTERNATIVE METHODS
Hair removal		++++	• Electroepilation • Waxing • Shaving
Wrinkle treatment		+++	• Chemical peeling • Mechanical dermabrasion • Dermal fillers and threads • Botulinum toxin type A (BTA) injection
Skin rejuve-nation	Laser derm-abrasion (predominantly age-related wrinkles)	+++ / ++++	• Chemical peeling • Mechanical dermabrasion • Dermal fillers and threads • BTA injection • Microneedling • Mesotherapy
	Fractional abla-tive treatment	++ / +++	• Dermal fillers and threads • Microneedling • RF microneedling
	Fractional non-ablative treatment	+ / ++	• Dermal fillers and threads • Chemical peeling • RF thermolifting
Treatment of vascular pathologies		+++ / ++++	• Electrocoagulation
Treatment of pigmentary pathologies		++ / +++ / ++++	• Chemical peeling • Topical depigmentants
Tattoo removal		++ / +++ / ++++	• Chemical disintegration • Laser resurfacing

++++ – high; +++ – moderate; ++ – low

Thus, it is possible to identify the so-called **basic laser services**, which is optimal in terms of efficiency and cost:

- Hair removal
- Rejuvenation — it is better to start with non-ablative laser treatment, which does not require an operating room and subsequent long rehabilitation (as an option: treatment of vascular and pigmentary pathology = photorejuvenation)
- Removal of skin growths

The following are considered **complementary laser services**:

- Laser rejuvenation (laser dermabrasion, fractional ablative photothermolysis)
- Scar revision, including post-acne
- Tattoo removal
- Aesthetic laser phlebology
- Laser lipolysis and liposuction
- Laser gynecology

2.2. What to look for when choosing laser equipment

Virtually any laser can be used to treat several different conditions by changing its operating parameters or combining it with other technologies. For example, PDL or Nd:YAG (main indications: vascular pathology, epilation) can be used for the removal of warts, keratosis, and stimulation of collagen synthesis in the periorbital zone, while ALEX (epilation) is well-suited for the correction of vascular and pigment defects. CO_2 laser is a multitasking device in general and when equipped with the appropriate probes can be used for the correction of photo- and chrono-aging signs, as well as scars and striae, eyelid lift, removal of formations (including pigmented), gynecological treatment, ear, nose, and throat (ENT) and dental pathologies, and so on.

Similar "broad spectrum of action" characterizes IPL devices, which, unlike lasers, produce radiation in a broadband spectrum (on average from 500 to 1200 nm), which is absorbed by various chromophores in the skin (hemoglobin, melanin, water).

In addition, a large number of multifunctional platforms are now available on the market, which can be equipped with different modules (different lasers, IPL, RF, etc.), gradually expanding the range of services based on just one device. For example, IPL beam is distributed to all targets in its path, so the deeper structures receive much less energy than in the case of lasers, due to which the efficiency of the procedures will be lower. However, modern IPL devices are approaching lasers in their parameters, which is the reason for their "second birth" observed in recent years.

Still, when choosing a device, it is necessary to pay attention not only to the technical parameters, but also to a number of other factors:

- Type of practice — skincare, dermatology, salon/spa, phlebology, plastic surgery
- Format of the medical center: a small center with one room, a center with two rooms (manipulation, procedure), a large center with laser specialization, mixed format — surgery + skincare
- Availability of rooms certified for laser equipment use
- Availability of operating room/procedure room for laser resurfacing, invasive procedures
- Availability of specialists with the appropriate skills and willingness to work with lasers
- Regional, including ethnic, characteristics
- Financial expectations — adequate business plan (or feasibility study), amount of investment, etc.

For example, buying a modern multifunctional CO_2 laser (based on distributors' advertising statements) in a mid-level clinic that does not have the conditions and license to perform surgical procedures will be comparable to buying a Lamborghini and driving it to the countryside. That is, return on investment in a particular device is limited by the inability to perform a certain volume of procedures, making such purchase financially imprudent. In addition, the same equipment allows practitioners to perform a different range of interventions. It is recommended to divide the pricing policy not only depending on the technical complexity of the procedure, but also on the solvency of patients. For example, the difference in cost between laser rejuvenation for mature patients who are willing to pay a high price for the procedure and post-acne scar resurfacing, which is in high demand among moneyless young people, will not raise any questions. Moreover, this approach can enhance the reputation of the center.

In order to avoid mistakes, it is necessary to carefully evaluate all aspects of the available practice. The following are recommendations for equipping different types of aesthetic facilities to ensure optimal work with laser equipment.

2.3. Beauty salons, spa/wellness centers, skincare offices

Features
- Predominance of treatment and injection procedures
- As a rule, these are start-ups and low-budget organizations
- No extra floor space
- Limited medical staff

Recommended procedures
- Non-invasive rejuvenation
- Non-invasive hair removal

Recommended devices
- First-line units:
  - IPL device is an optimal choice because the availability of various filters allows practitioners to perform photoepilation, as well as removal of vascular and pigmented lesions, along with stimulation of collagen synthesis (i.e., photorejuvenation). Not all IPL devices are equally good, as not every device can produce several consecutive pulses as well as change the energy density regardless of the pulse duration; the lack of such a possibility reduces the effectiveness of selective action on vascular or pigmented structures.
  - Vascular lasers (KTP, PDL, Nd:YAG) are an alternative to the first option (removal of vascular defects is the third most

popular laser procedure after hair removal and rejuvenation). They are much more effective in removing telangiectasias and lentigos and can smooth wrinkles but do not remove hair.

- Devices of the second stage:
  - RF devices (including RF microneedling)
  - Gas–liquid peeling device
  - High-intensity focused ultrasound (HIFU) device

2.4. Small medical centers

Features
- One room for a laser device
- 1–2 qualified operators

Recommended procedures
- Epilation
- Non-invasive rejuvenation
- Acne treatment
- Onychomycosis treatment
- Body shaping
- Vascular lesion coagulation

Recommended devices
- First-line units

The optimal choice will be a multifunctional platform with the possibility of purchasing additional probes.

Basic probes:
- IPL: removal of blood vessels, pigment, hair
- Epilation laser: ALEX, Diode
- Non-invasive rejuvenation: non-ablative fractional photothermolysis, RF microneedling

Optional probes:
- Ablative fractional probe for rejuvenation: Er:YAG, CO_2
- Aesthetic phlebology, onychomycosis, acne: Nd:YAG

- Devices of the second stage:
  - For laser-associated liposuction (minimally invasive lipolysis)
  - For endovenous photocoagulation for the treatment of varicose veins
  - For removing neoplasms: e.g., RF electrocoagulator

Laser-assisted liposuction and endovenous laser photocoagulation require an operating room, surgeons, post-operative rooms, and a surgical license.

2.5. Medium-sized medical centers

Features
- Availability of manipulation and procedure rooms (for invasive procedures)
- Availability of several qualified specialists

Recommended devices
- General skincare practice:
  - Manipulation room — a multifunctional platform or an IPL device. Specialization in the provision of selected medical services:
    1) epilation: the first-line device — ALEX laser (quickly creates demand for the service), the second-line device — Diode laser (to expand the service, it is possible to perform epilation for I–V phototypes)
    2) vascular disorders: KTP, PDL, Nd:YAG/KTP
    3) rejuvenation, acne treatment, onychomycosis: ALEX/Nd:YAG
  - Procedure room — multitasking CO_2 laser with probes for surgery, continuous ablation, and fractional phototermolysis

- Second stage devices (optional):
  - Laser for fractional photothermolysis: photoaging treatment, anti-aging treatment (well combined with IPL and vascular lasers)

- QS laser for tattoo removal and pigmentation treatment
- Gynecologic CO_2 or Erbium laser probe (if there is a gynecologic service)
- Devices for endovenous laser photocoagulation (if an operating room is available)
- Lasers for photodynamic therapy (acne treatment, rejuvenation, rehabilitation, etc.)
- Excimer laser for treatment of psoriasis, vitiligo (expensive equipment, but justified for certain regions and federal institutions)

Attention: Trained qualified personnel is mandatory!

2.6. Medical centers with mixed practice: skincare, dermatology, and plastic surgery

Features
- Number of rooms — at least three
- Separation of flows and pricing policies

Recommended procedures and devices
- Skincare services:
  - Laser for hair removal
  - IPL
  - Laser for fractional photothermolysis
- Dermatology services:
  - CO_2 or Erbium lasers (scars and stretch marks revision, neoplasms removal)
  - Vascular laser (removal of vascular formations, including varicose veins)
  - Lasers for the treatment of acne (including PDT)
  - QS lasers for the removal of tattoos and pigmented lesions
- Plastic surgery + cosmetic dermatology:
  - CO_2 laser is a must. The optimal choice is an ultrashort-pulsed CO_2 laser with all probes — for continuous ablation (resurfacing), fractional superficial, fractional deep treatment, etc.

The device allows clinicians not only to perform, but also qualitatively complement certain types of surgical interventions, such as laser skin resurfacing + surgical skin tightening, transconjunctival blepharoplasty + laser skin tightening, elimination of excess skin after rhinoplasty, scar revision after plastic surgery, and laser eyelid skin tightening as an addition or correction after blepharoplasty.
- Vascular lasers (PDL, KTP) can be used to treat fresh scars, remove telangiectasias after plastic surgery and filler injections, improve skin texture and elasticity, and treat erythema after deep laser resurfacing.

2.7. Centers of expert level

A center of expert level implies a wide range of services. At the same time, one should expect that laser hair removal procedures, rejuvenation, and elimination of vascular pathology will still generate the main profit. However, it is the provision of exclusive services that will justify device purchases for this category of institution.

Features: positioning of the institution as a specialized center for laser cosmetic dermatology and surgery or, alternatively, a center for laser correction of congenital and acquired skin defects.

Recommended procedures and devices
- Age-related changes and photoaging: ultrashort-pulsed CO_2, Er:YAG, picosecond QS laser with fractional probe
- Epilation: ALEX, Diode
- Vascular lesions: PDL/Nd:YAG, KTP
- Pigment lesions, tattoo removal: QS laser (picosecond), CO_2
- Phlebology: Nd:YAG + laser for endovenous photocoagulation
- Acne treatment: vascular lasers, CO_2, PDT
- Body shaping, cellulite treatment: lipolysis laser with special probes (1064, 1320, 1440 nm)
- Gynecology: CO_2, Er:YAG with special probes
- Fungal lesions: Nd:YAG
- Psoriasis, vitiligo: Excimer laser

2.8. Challenges of laser-based practice

Problems associated with using laser equipment can be divided into two types: those that are inevitable and those the occurrence of which can be corrected.

The first type includes:
- High cost of equipment
- The need to replace consumable parts in some types of devices, which will increase the treatment cost
- Strict regulations on the safety of use

Lasers used in cosmetic dermatology practice are hazard devices of the III–IV class. They require separate rooms, safety systems (goggles, smoke evacuator), and other work equipment. **Table III-2-2** summarizes the basic requirements for laser rooms.

Table III-2-2. Basic requirements for laser rooms

ROOM ELEMENT	REQUIREMENTS
Office	The area shall not be less than 12 m² in size. The doors to the room should be equipped with an external signboard LASER AREA, DO NOT ENTER, a laser hazard sign, and an internal locking device.
Walls	Coating — easy to clean, light-colored, matte finish.
Floor	Of non-combustible, laser-absorbing and electrically insulating material, also light-colored and frosted.
Elements of design	There should be no mirrored surfaces in the room and windows should have non-glossy blinds or non-flammable curtains.
Ventilation	If necessary, the workplace shall be equipped with local exhaust ventilation to remove combustion products.
Protection	Both operator and patient must wear protective goggles during laser session. If necessary, a smoke vent should be used.

The second type of possible problems includes:

- Risks of complications such as burns, scars, hyper- or hypopigmentation, etc. (continuous professional development of personnel, proper selection of patients, selection of adequate treatment parameters, and compliance with technical and safety regulations contribute to risk reduction).
- Financial risks associated with incorrect center positioning, choice of equipment, and, consequently, provision of services.
- Professionals' fears of lasers, low competence of personnel and, consequently, inadequate provision of information to the patient, which reduces the number of prescriptions for laser procedures or leads to their replacement by alternative methods, but with much less specificity of action and clinical effect.
- The owner's desire to turn all specialists into "multi-taskers" leads to a shortage or excess of target services — the principle of "what is easier for me to sell, I will provide..." begins to work.

2.9. Optimization of laser center operation

Today, there is a tendency towards narrow specialization, giving rise to a wide variety of "laser specialists" — skincare practitioners, phlebologists, oncologists, surgeons, etc. — who mainly use lasers as a tool. A positive aspect of such laser specialization is that practitioners are concentrated on and interested in using lasers. As a result, they are better able to "sell" these services and are motivated to improve their knowledge and experience, expand their practice, learn new methods, etc.

However, it is important not only to improve the qualifications of doctors, but also to train administrators to sell laser services. Administrators are the first staff members clients encounter, so their attitude and knowledge will determine whether the client reaches the doctor. Therefore, they must be able to describe the service in such a way that patients will want to buy it. Proper marketing of services — positioning laser procedures as high-tech medical care — is also important. According to the current legislation, neither injectable cosmetology nor plastic surgery (except auxiliary aids) are classified as high-tech medical care, unlike lasers. This needs to be emphasized.

A separate point of optimization concerns the choice of laser equipment itself. First, devices should be purchased only from well-known brands with quality service from distribution companies. Second, when making such purchase, regional peculiarities should be considered. For example, in the southern regions, there is a high incidence of pigmentary disorders, which justifies the purchase of devices that can be used to treat this pathology. Diode or Nd:YAG lasers are more suitable for hair removal in this region. Practitioners should also be careful with the use of CO_2 laser (and may opt for Er:YAG as an alternative). Conversely, in northern latitudes, where it is windy and there are large temperature variations, there is a high percentage of patients with telangiectasias (couperosis). Consequently, we can predict a high demand for "vascular" lasers in this case.

Thus, as mentioned above, a good optimization option is to conduct price diversification, as this strategy will allow the practice to reach a more significant market segment by attracting the greatest number of potential consumers with different financial capabilities.

Lasers are complex and expensive devices, and their performance is affected by various factors. Many of these are of human origin and can be optimized.

Failure to use laser technology in one's practice leads to a considerable loss of benefits. Worldwide, there is an annual increase in the popularity of device-based interventions, and the share of lasers among them is predominant. There is a website, www.realself.com, which collects consumer reviews (tens of thousands of reviews) on various aesthetic procedures and specific devices and preparations. Users can express their opinions in two ways — they can recommend this service to others or warn them against it. For laser procedures, consistently high results are reported. For example, 83% of clients recommend fractional laser rejuvenation using CO_2 laser, while, for example, for superficial musculo-aponeurotic system (SMAS) lifting procedure with focused ultrasound, this figure is about 60%. Thus, the availability of laser technologies in practice will help raise it to a higher level, and a conscious choice of devices will help make the work with them as effective as possible.

References

Ablon G. Phototherapy with light emitting diodes: treating a broad range of medical and aesthetic conditions in dermatology. J Clin Aesthet Dermatol 2018; 11(2): 21–27.

Alster T.S., Li M.K. Dermatologic laser side effects and complications: prevention and management. Am J Clin Dermatol 2020; 21(5): 711–723.

Altshuler G.B., Anderson R.R., Manstein D. et al. Extended theory of selective photothermolysis. Lasers Surg Med 2001; 29(5): 416–432.

Alyoussef A. Excimer laser system: the revolutionary way to treat psoriasis. Cureus 2023; 15(12): e50249.

Amini-Nik S., Kraemer D., Cowan M.L. et al. Ultrafast mid-IR laser scalpel: protein signals of the fundamental limits to minimally invasive surgery. PLoS One 2010; 5(9): e13053.

Anderson R.R. Lasers for dermatology and skin biology. J Invest Dermatol 2013; 133(E1): E21–E23.

Anderson R.R., Parrish J.A. Selective photothermolysis: precise microsurgery by selective absorption of pulsed radiation. Science 1983; 220(4596): 524–527.

Araghi F., Ohadi L., Moravvej H. et al. Laser treatment of benign melanocytic lesion: a review. Lasers Med Sci 2022; 37(9): 3353–3362.

Ardeleanu V., Radaschin S.D., Tatu A.L. Excimer laser for psoriasis treatment: a case report and short review. Exp Ther Med 2020; 20(1): 52–55.

Avci P., Gupta A., Sadasivam M. et al. Low-level laser (light) therapy (LLLT) in skin: stimulating, healing, restoring. Semin Cutan Med Surg 2013b; 32(1): 41–52.

Avci P., Nyame T.T., Gupta G.K. et al. Low-level laser therapy for fat layer reduction: a comprehensive review. Lasers Surg Med 2013a; 45(6): 349–357.

Barbaric J., Abbott R., Posadzki P. et al. Light therapies for acne. Cochrane Database Syst Rev 2016; 9(9): CD007917.

Bernabe R.M., Choe D., Calero T. et al. Laser-assisted drug delivery in the treatment of hypertrophic scars and keloids: a systematic review. J Burn Care Res 2024; irae023.

Bernestein L.J., Geronemus R.G. Keloid formation with the 585-nm pulsed dye laser during isotretinoin treatment. Arch Dermatol 1997; 133(1): 111–112.

Boehm K.S., Avashia Y.J., Savetsky I.L., Rohrich R.J. Laser resurfacing: safety and technique. Plast Reconstr Surg Glob Open 2020; 8(4): e2796.

Bragina I.Y. Combination of hyaluronic-based fillers and physiotherapeutic technologies in one treatment zone. Injection Methods in Cosmetology 2018; 1: 102–109.

Castano A.P., Demidova T.N., Hamblin M.R. Mechanisms in photodynamic therapy. Part 1: photosensitizers, photochemistry and cellular localization. Photodiagnosis Photodyn Ther 2004; 1: 279–293.

Chen S.X., Cheng J., Watchmaker J. et al. Review of lasers and energy-based devices for skin rejuvenation and scar treatment with histologic correlations. Dermatol Surg 2022; 48(4): 441–448.

Chu G.Y., Huang C.C., Shih N.H. et al. The 1450-nm diode laser reduces redness and porphyrin density: an image-based, patient-oriented appraisal. J Clin Med 2023; 12(13): 4500.

Couturaud V., Le Fur M., Pelletier M., Granotier F. Reverse skin aging signs by red light photobiomodulation. Skin Res Technol 2023; 29(7): e13391.

Dai X., Jin S., Xuan Y. et al. 590 nm LED irradiation improved erythema through inhibiting angiogenesis of human microvascular endothelial cells and ameliorated pigmentation in melasma. Cells 2022; 11(24): 3949.

Darlenski R., Fluhr J.W. Photodynamic therapy in dermatology: past, present, and future. J Biomed Opt 2013; 18(6): 061208.

DiBernardo B.E., Pozner J.N. Intense pulsed light therapy for skin rejuvenation. Clin Plast Surg 2016; 43(3): 535–540.

Diogo M.L.G., Campos T.M., Fonseca E.S.R. et al. Effect of blue light on acne vulgaris: a systematic review. Sensors (Basel) 2021; 21(20): 6943.

Doppegieter M., van der Beek N., Bakker E.N.T.P. et al. Effects of pulsed dye laser treatment in psoriasis: a nerve-wrecking process? Exp Dermatol 2023; 32(7): 1165–1173.

Dorgham N.A., Dorgham D.A. Lasers for reduction of unwanted hair in skin of colour: a systematic review and meta-analysis. J Eur Acad Dermatol Venereol 2020; 34(5): 948–955.

Eichler H.J., Eichler J., Lux O. Lasers. Basics, advances and applications. Springer Series in Optical Sciences (SSOS, volume 220). Springer, 2018.

Farkas J.P., Hoopman J.E., Kenkel J.M. Five parameters you must understand to master control of your laser/light-based devices. Aesthet Surg J 2013; (7): 1059–1064.

Farkas J.P., Richardson J.A., Brown S. et al. Effects of common laser treatments on hyaluronic acid fillers in a porcine model. Aesthet Surg J 2008; 28(5): 503–511.

Fayne R.A., Perper M., Eber A.E. et al. Laser and light treatments for hair reduction in Fitzpatrick skin types IV-VI: a comprehensive review of the literature. Am J Clin Dermatol 2018; 19(2): 237–252.

Fernandez-Nieto D., Jimenez-Cauhe J., Ortega-Quijano D., Boixeda P. A novel high-power 1060-nm diode laser for the treatment of vascular malformations: a pilot study using dermoscopy to evaluate clinical endpoints. Lasers Med Sci 2021; 36(2): 455–461.

Friedman D.J. Successful treatment of a red and black professional tattoo in skin type VI with a picosecond dual-wavelength, neodymium-doped yttrium aluminium garnet laser. Dermatol Surg 2016; 42(9): 1121–1123.

Gade A., Vasile G.F., Rubenstein R. Intense pulsed light (IPL) therapy. StatPearls [Internet], 2023; StatPearls Publishing, 2024.

Gaffey M.M., Johnson A.B. Laser treatment of pigmented lesions. StatPearls [Internet], 2023; StatPearls Publishing, 2024.

Giovanni C., Marina P.B., Tiziano Z. A retrospective 10-years-experience overview of dye laser treatments for vascular pathologies. Skin Res Technol 2023; 29(8): e13427.

Gloviczki P., Lawrence P.F., Wasan S.M. et al. The 2022 Society for Vascular Surgery, American Venous Forum, and American Vein and Lymphatic Society clinical practice guidelines for the management of varicose veins of the lower extremities. Part I. Duplex scanning and treatment of superficial truncal reflux: endorsed by the Society for Vascular Medicine and the International Union of Phlebology. J Vasc Surg Venous Lymphat Disord 2023; 11(2): 231–261.

Gold M.H., Weiss E., Biron J. Novel laser hair removal in all skin types. J Cosmet Dermatol 2023; 22(4): 1261–1265.

Goldman L., Wilson R.G., Hornby P., Meyer R.G. Radiation from a Q-switched ruby laser. Effect of repeated impacts of power output of 10 megawatts on a tattoo of man. J Invest Dermatol 1965; 44: 69–71.

Goldman M.P., Alster T.S., Weiss R. A randomized trial to determine the influence of laser therapy, monopolar radiofrequency treatment, and intense pulsed light therapy administered immediately after hyaluronic acid gel implantation. Dermatol Surg 2007; 33(5): 535–542.

Hamblin M.R. Photobiomodulation or low-level laser therapy. J Biophotonics 2016; 9(11–12): 1122–1124.

Han G. Basics of lasers in dermatology. Cutis 2014; 94(3): E23–E25.

Heidari Beigvand H., Razzaghi M., Rostami-Nejad M. et al. Assessment of laser effects on skin rejuvenation. J Lasers Med Sci 2020; 11(2): 212–219.

Hernandez L., Mohsin N., Frech F.S. et al. Laser tattoo removal: laser principles and an updated guide for clinicians. Lasers Med Sci 2022; 37(6): 2581–2587.

Hsiao C.Y., Yang S.C., Alalaiwe A., Fang J.Y. Laser ablation and topical drug delivery: a review of recent advances. Expert Opin Drug Deliv 2019; 16(9): 937–952.

Hsu S.H., Chung H.J., Weiss R.A. Histologic effects of fractional laser and radiofrequency devices on hyaluronic acid filler. Dermatol Surg 2019; 45(4): 552–556.

Hügül H., Özkoca D., Kirişci M., Kutlubay Z. Treatment indications of carbon solution-assisted Nd:YAG laser according to patient satisfaction: a retrospective study. Dermatol Pract Concept 2023; 13(4): e2023219.

Husain Z., Alster T.S. The role of lasers and intense pulsed light technology in dermatology. Clin Cosmet Investig Dermatol 2016; 9: 29–40.

Jih M.H., Kimyai-Asadi A. Laser treatment of acne vulgaris. Semin Plast Surg 2007; 21(3): 167–174.

Kalashnikova N.G., Jafferany M., Lotti T. Management and prevention of laser complications in aesthetic medicine: analysis of the etiological factors. Dermatol Ther 2021; 34(1): e14373.

Kang C.N., Shah M., Lynde C., Fleming P. Hair removal practices: a literature review. Skin Therapy Lett 2021; 26(5): 6–11.

Knight J.M., Kautz G. Sequential facial skin rejuvenation with intense pulsed light and non-ablative fractionated laser resurfacing in Fitzpatrick skin type II–IV patients: a prospective multicenter analysis. Lasers Surg Med 2019; 51(2): 141–149.

Ko D., Wang R.F., Ozog D. et al. Disorders of hyperpigmentation. Part II. Review of management and treatment options for hyperpigmentation. J Am Acad Dermatol 2023; 88(2): 291–320.

Kurniadi I., Tabri F., Madjid A. et al. Laser tattoo removal: fundamental principles and practical approach. Dermatol Ther 2021; 34(1): e14418.

Lai D., Zhou S., Cheng S. et al. Laser therapy in the treatment of melasma: a systematic review and meta-analysis. Lasers Med Sci 2022; 37(4): 2099–2110.

Laubach H.J., Tannous Z., Anderson R.R., Manstein D. Skin responses to fractional photothermolysis. Lasers Surg Med 2006; 38(2): 142–149.

Lee C.M. Laser-assisted hair removal for facial hirsutism in women: a review of evidence. J Cosmet Laser Ther 2018; 20(3): 140–144.

Lee C.N., Hsu R., Chen H., Wong T.W. Daylight photodynamic therapy: an update. Molecules 2020; 25(21): 5195.

Lee J.Y., Oh S.W., Ryu H.Y., Seo Y.S. Development of a minimally invasive and non-invasive lipolysis laser system for effective fat reduction. J Lasers Med Sci 2021; 12: e55.

Leszczynski R., da Silva C.A., Pinto A.C.P.N. et al. Laser therapy for treating hypertrophic and keloid scars. Cochrane Database Syst Rev 2022; 9(9): CD011642.

Leu F.J., Huang C.L., Wu Y.S., Wang C.C. Comparison of picosecond versus nanosecond Nd:YAG lasers for the removal of cosmetic tattoos in an animal model. Lasers Med Sci 2022; 37(2): 1343–1350.

Lin C.H., Aljuffali I.A., Fang J.Y. Lasers as an approach for promoting drug delivery via skin. Expert Opin Drug Deliv 2014; 11(4): 599–614.

Li Pomi F., Vaccaro M., Peterle L., Borgia F. Photodynamic therapy for severe acne. Photodiagnosis Photodyn Ther 2024; 45: 103893.

Manstein D., Herron G.S., Sink R.K. et al. Fractional photothermolysis: a new concept for cutaneous remodeling using microscopic patterns of thermal injury. Lasers Surg Med 2004; 34(5): 426–438.

Maranda E.L., Lim V.M., Nguyen A.H., Nouri K. Laser and light therapy for facial warts: a systematic review. J Eur Acad Dermatol Venereol 2016; 30(10): 1700–1707.

Meesters A.A., De Rie M.A., Wolkerstorfer A. Generalized eczematous reaction after fractional carbon dioxide laser therapy for tattoo allergy. J Cosmet Laser Ther 2016; 18(8): 456–458.

Mollet I., Ongenae K., Naeyaert J.M. Origin, clinical presentation, and diagnosis of hypomelanotic skin disorders. Dermatol Clin 2007; 25(3): 363–371, ix.

Moskvin S.V. Low-level laser therapy: "Western school" vs "Eastern school." J Lasers Med Sci 2021; 12: e66.

Munavalli G. Photopneumatic technology for the treatment of mild-to-moderate acne vulgaris – a review. J Clin Aesthet Dermatol 2023; 16(6 Suppl 2): S4–S6.

Murphy M.J., Torstensson PA. Thermal relaxation times: an outdated concept in photothermal treatments. Lasers Med Sci 2014; 29(3): 973–978.

Mysore V., Omprakash H.M., Khatri G.N. Isotretinoin and dermatosurgical procedures. Indian J Dermatol Venereol Leprol 2019; 85(1): 18–23.

Nabi N., Bhat Y.J., Dar U.K. et al. Comparative study of the clinico-trichoscopic response to treatment of hirsutism with long pulsed (1064 nm) Nd:YAG laser in idiopathic hirsutism and polycystic ovarian syndrome patients. Lasers Med Sci 2022; 37(1): 545–553.

Nestor M., Andriessen A., Berman B. et al. Photobiomodulation with non-thermal lasers: mechanisms of action and therapeutic uses in dermatology and aesthetic medicine. J Cosmet Laser Ther 2017; 19(4): 190–198.

Niemz M.H. Laser–tissue Interactions: Fundamentals and Applications, 4th ed. Springer, 2019.

Nouri K. (ed.). Lasers in Dermatology and Medicine, 2nd ed. Springer, 2012.

Omi T., Numano K. The Role of the CO_2 laser and fractional CO_2 laser in dermatology. Laser Ther 2014; 23(1): 49–60.

Orringer J.S., Kang S., Johnson T.M. et al. Connective tissue remodeling induced by carbon dioxide laser resurfacing of photodamaged human skin. Arch Dermatol 2004; 140(11): 1326–1332.

Park K.Y., Park M.K., Li K. et al. Combined treatment with a non-ablative infrared device and hyaluronic acid filler does not have enhanced efficacy in treating nasolabial fold wrinkles. Dermatol Surg 2011; 37(12): 1770–1775.

Piccolo D., Pieri L., Fusco I. et al. Removal of unwanted hair: efficacy and safety of 755-nm alexandrite laser equipped with a 30 mm spot handpiece. Photobiomodul Photomed Laser Surg 2023; 41(9): 509–511.

Post N.F., Ezekwe N., Narayan V.S. et al. The use of lasers in vitiligo, an overview. J Eur Acad Dermatol Venereol 2022; 36(6): 779–789.

Prather H.B., Alam M., Poon E. et al. Laser safety in isotretinoin use: a survey of expert opinion and practice. Dermatol Surg 2017; 43(3): 357–363.

Rajabi-Estarabadi A., Choragudi S., Camacho I. et al. Effectiveness of photopneumatic technology: a descriptive review of the literature. Lasers Med Sci 2018; 33(8): 1631–1637.

Reddy K.K., Brauer J.A., Anolik R. et al. Topical perfluorodecalin resolves immediate whitening reactions and allows rapid effective multiple pass treatment of tattoos. Lasers Surg Med 2013; 45(2): 76–80.

Ribé A., Ribé N. Neck skin rejuvenation: histological and clinical changes after combined therapy with a fractional non-ablative laser and stabilized hyaluronic acid-based gel of non-animal origin. J Cosmet Laser Ther 2001; 13(4): 154–161.

Rkein A.M., Ozog D.M. Photodynamic therapy. Dermatol Clin 2014; 32(3): 415–425.

Ross E.V. Extended theory of selective photothermolysis: a new recipe for hair cooking? Lasers Surg Med 2001; 29(5): 413–415.

Sadowska M., Narbutt J., Lesiak A. Blue light in dermatology. Life (Basel) 2021; 11(7): 670.

Sales A.F.S., Pandolfo I.L., de Almeida Cruz M. et al. Intense pulsed light on skin rejuvenation: a systematic review. Arch Dermatol Res 2022; 314(9): 823–838.

Sapra S., Lultschik S.D., Tran J.V., Dong K. Concomitant therapy of oral isotretinoin with multiplex pulsed dye laser and Nd:YAG laser for acne. J Clin Aesthet Dermatol 2022; 15(9): 20–24.

Schilling L., Saedi N., Weiss R. 1060 nm diode hyperthermic laser lipolysis: the latest in non-invasive body contouring. J Drugs Dermatol 2017; 16(1): 48–52.

Schreiver I., Hutzler C., Andree S. et al. Identification and hazard prediction of tattoo pigments by means of pyrolysis–gas chromatography/mass spectrometry. Arch Toxicol 2016; 90(7): 1639–1650.

Sheptii O.V. Laser therapy of vascular skin pathology: basic principles and practical recommendations. Apparatnaya Kosmetologia 2018; 1–2: 54–66.

Snast I., Kaftory R., Lapidoth M., Levi A. Paradoxical hypertrichosis associated with laser and light therapy for hair removal: a systematic review and meta-analysis. Am J Clin Dermatol 2021; 22(5): 615–624.

Terra Garcia M., Correia Pereira A.H., Figueiredo-Godoi L.M.A. et al. Photodynamic therapy mediated by chlorin-type photosensitizers against Streptococcus mutans biofilms. Photodiagnosis Photodyn Ther 2018; 24: 256–261.

Trelles M.A., Khomchenko V., Alcolea J.M., Martínez-Carpio P.A. A novel method of facial rejuvenation using a 2940-nm Er:YAG laser with spatially modulated ablation: a pilot study. Lasers Med Sci 2016; 31(7): 1465–1471.

Urdiales-Gálvez F., Martin-Sánchez S., Maíz-Jiménez M. et al. Concomitant use of hyaluronic acid and laser in facial rejuvenation. Aesthetic Plast Surg 2019; 43(4): 1061–1070.

van Zuuren E.J., Arents B.W.M., van der Linden M.M.D. et al. Rosacea: new concepts in classification and treatment. Am J Clin Dermatol 2021; 22(4): 457–465.

Verma N., Yumeen S., Raggio B.S. Ablative laser resurfacing. StatPearls [Internet], 2023; StatPearls Publishing, 2024.

Volkova N.V., Valamina I.E., Shvidun D.V. et al. Facial rejuvenation using Er:YAG laser equipped with a spatially modulated ablation module: a clinical, ultrasound, and histological evaluation. J Cosmet Dermatol 2019; 18(5): 1294–1299.

Waldman A., Bolotin D., Arndt K.A. et al. ASDS guidelines task force: consensus recommendations regarding the safety of lasers, dermabrasion, chemical peels, energy devices, and skin surgery during and after isotretinoin use. Dermatol Surg 2017; 43(10): 1249–1262.

Wang D., Yan Y., Wang P. et al. A prospective, split-face, randomized controlled trial of intense pulsed light-photodynamic therapy for seborrhea. Photodiagnosis Photodyn Ther 2024; 45: 103973.

Wang R.F., Ko D., Friedman B.J. et al. Disorders of hyperpigmentation. Part I. Pathogenesis and clinical features of common pigmentary disorders. J Am Acad Dermatol 2023; 88(2): 271–288.

Wenande E., Erlendsson A.M., Haedersdal M. Opportunities for laser-assisted drug delivery in the treatment of cutaneous disorders. Semin Cutan Med Surg 2017; 36(4): 192–201.

Willardson H.B., Kobayashi T.T., Arnold J.G. et al. Diffuse urticarial reaction associated with titanium dioxide following laser tattoo removal treatments. Photomed Laser Surg 2017; 35(3): 176–180.

Wollina U. Seborrheic keratoses — the most common benign skin tumor of humans. Clinical presentation and an update on pathogenesis and treatment options. Open Access Maced J Med Sci 2018; 6(11): 2270–2275.

Wu X., Wang X., Wu X. et al. Intense pulsed light therapy improves acne-induced postinflammatory erythema and hyperpigmentation: a retrospective study in Chinese patients. Dermatol Ther (Heidelb) 2022; 12(5): 1147–1156.

Xiao A., Ettefagh L. Laser Revision of Scars. StatPearls [Internet], 2022; StatPearls Publishing, 2024.

Ying Z.X., Zhao Y.B., Li D. et al. The influence of morphological distribution of melanin on parameter selection in laser thermotherapy for vascular skin diseases. Lasers Med Sci 2020; 35(4): 901–917.

Yumeen S., Hohman M.H., Khan T. Laser Er:YAG resurfacing. StatPearls [Internet], 2023; StatPearls Publishing, 2024.

Yumeen S., Khan T. Laser carbon dioxide resurfacing. StatPearls [Internet], 2023; StatPearls Publishing, 2024.

Zhang C., Lyu W., Qiu P. et al. Laser ablation on vascular diseases: mechanisms and influencing factors. Lasers Med Sci 2023; 39(1): 18.

Zhang J., Duan J., Gong L. Super pulse CO_2 laser therapy for benign eyelid tumors. J Cosmet Dermatol 2018; 17(2): 171–175.

Zhang P., Wu M.X. A clinical review of phototherapy for psoriasis. Lasers Med Sci 2018; 33(1): 173–180.

Zhang Y., Jiang S., Lu Y. et al. A decade retrospective study of light/laser devices in treating nasal rosacea. J Dermatolog Treat 2020; 31(1): 84–90.

www.ingramcontent.com/pod-product-compliance
Lightning Source LLC
Chambersburg PA
CBHW052018030426
42335CB00026B/3189